IN THE COMPANY OF GRACE

IN THE COMPANY OF GRACE

A VETERINARIAN'S MEMOIR OF TRAUMA AND HEALING

Jody Lulich

UNIVERSITY OF MINNESOTA PRESS
MINNEAPOLIS
LONDON

Published by the University of Minnesota Press
111 Third Avenue South, Suite 290
Minneapolis, MN 55401-2520
http://www.upress.umn.edu

ISBN 978-1-5179-1419-6 (pb)

A Cataloging-in-Publication record for this book is
available from the Library of Congress.

Printed in the United States of America on acid-free paper

The University of Minnesota is an
equal-opportunity educator and employer.

31 30 29 28 27 26 25 24 23   10 9 8 7 6 5 4 3 2 1

To Grace P. Hooks

And to all the mothers and fathers, whether blood-related or not, who parented me with love, tenderness, patience, and understanding: Betty Jean Lulich, Joseph Lulich, Ora Lee Davis, Jessie Galvin, Bobbie and Julia Bell, Ethel Thames, Charlotte Paglin, Donice Daigre, Thelma Murphy, Jannetta and Bruce Yancey, Thomas Wake, Carl Osborne, Edith Calhoun, Uncles Marty and Buddy, Aunts Cleo, Joyce, Kathy, Shirley, and Beverly, and Joseph Lhm.

There's a crack in everything, that's how the light gets in.
—LEONARD COHEN

CONTENTS

PROLOGUE

As the lights went down over the audience and up on the stage, my heart raced. And not in a good way.

I was one of several veterinarians being honored that evening. I sat in the front row in a dark-blue suit, starched white shirt, and blue tie. The room was cold, but I was overheating. My eyeglasses fogged over. I squinted, but could only make out hazy beams of white light fanning down from the ceiling to the stage floor. I shifted my arms away from the sides of my body to dissipate the heat. I took off my glasses and wiped them clean. I turned around and looked behind me. Every seat in the auditorium was filled.

Many in the audience I knew. And many of them thought they knew me.

In my hand, I held a single sheet of paper. On one side, I had written the speech I wanted to tell—*I became a veterinarian because the doctor who cared for my sick dog was gentle and patient. At a young age, I knew I wanted to be just like him.*

On the other side, I had written the speech I needed to tell—*When I was a little boy, my mother committed suicide. As my father drove to the funeral, a dog darted out from an alley. He ran in our direction. It was an accident, but our car hit him. The crumpling sound as the tires ran over its body jolted me hard against the back of the passenger seat. I squeezed my eyes shut and slowly lowered my head into my hands because I could have prevented it.*

I was torn between my past and the present, between what I was expected to say and how I became the man I am today. I no longer wanted to lie. But ashamed of the truth, I told no one.

I turned the paper over and over. Which speech do I tell? I needed to decide soon before my name was called.

FOUR WEEKS EARLIER, at work, my cell phone had rung. It was Dan, a colleague and friend. "Are you sitting down?" he asked.

"No, I'm at work."

"Then you should be sitting down. I'm calling because you've just been awarded the Morris Lifetime Achievement Award."

I chuckled. "Lifetime? Well, that makes me feel old."

He laughed and continued, "The award is presented to a veterinarian who has made significant contributions to the health and well-being of companion animals through a lifetime of service." It sounded like he was reading from a script. Then he ended with "Jody, this is a great honor."

I politely responded. "Wow, you're right, it is a great honor."

Dan described how pleased he was that I was the recipient. Then he told me the real reason for his call. "Jody, I've heard that you don't show up to accept awards."

He was right. I had not shown up to receive several teaching awards I'd been given over the years. I did not show up when my veterinary school presented me with the Distinguished Alumnus award fifteen years after my graduation.

"Jody, I'm calling because I want you to be there. The ceremony will be in Orlando, Florida, in a month. You can tell the audience what inspired you."

My lips parted and air rushed out. But I could not say out loud what I was thinking.

Dan emphasized that the award would cover all my expenses. Then he asked me again, "Jody, will you be there?"

During our conversation, I had been walking to the front of the hospital to see my first patient. Before reaching the lobby, I stopped. I focused on Dan's question. *Will I be there?*

Leaving freezing Minnesota in January for warmer weather in Florida sounded appealing. But for me, it was more about bringing up the past and dealing with my self-worth—two aspects of my life I desperately avoided. The days between Christmas and the first of the year were always difficult for me, as my mother had died early in the morning on the second of January, forty-five years ago.

Sure, I could graciously accept the award and walk away as if it would not affect me. Or I could tell the truth. I whispered to myself, "Do you really know the truth?" Both of my parents were dead, and the answers to many of my questions were buried with them. But I knew enough. Telling what I knew was my only way out.

As Dan went on talking about the award and the ceremony, I fell back into one of the chairs in the lobby. My backside slid forward and my legs twisted and folded in whatever position they landed. Bent up and unsupported, the way I felt my entire life.

Here I go again, I thought. I should feel grateful. But at times, I hated my job. I hated my life. I hadn't run over that dog. My father did. But the reason he was driving and the reason my mother was dead were partly my fault. And because of what happened, I was getting an award for a career that at times I considered more an obligation than a passion—a restitution that I often regretted more than enjoyed. And after all that I'd accomplished to make it right, my father had never put his arms around me, never looked me in the eye, and never said "Son, good job," or "way to go," or "I'm proud of you." If he was proud of me, he had a strange way of showing it.

I noticed that the phone was silent. I hoped that Dan had not been waiting long for my answer. I told myself that all I need to do is receive the award and say *Thank You.*

I sat up in the chair. Straightened my tie. Buttoned my lab coat. "Dan, you can count on it. I'll be there."

*

As I completed this book, my city was on fire. Protesters outraged over the murder of George Floyd by the Minneapolis police first demanded justice and later that evening took revenge. An estimated one thousand buildings across the Twin Cities were scorched: a barbershop, a pharmacy, a day care center, a dentist's office, a clothing store, an

Ethiopian restaurant, a post office, a police precinct, and many more.

Floyd, an unarmed Black man, should not have died. Police handcuffed him, forced him to the ground, turned him on his belly, and put their knees on his neck and back. He pleaded for mercy. *I can't breathe,* he said. Bystanders begged the police to get off George. *He can't breathe,* they shouted. *Get off him; he is struggling to breathe. Get off; he's unresponsive.* The crowd pleaded for mercy. The police did not waver. They held in place until George was dead, asphyxiated under the pressure of an officer's knee. The entire catastrophe, caught on a cell phone video, spread like wildfire. The injustice stunned the world, and the world erupted. And my city burned.

It was not the first time my city was burning. After the assassination of Martin Luther King Jr. in April 1968, the fires were so close to my home in Chicago that the smoke burned my eyes and the sounds of gunfire kept me awake at night. The unrest in Minneapolis that summer looked similar to what I had experienced then.

My parents met at a civil rights rally that turned into a riot. My father was struck in the head with an empty beer bottle, but what struck him most was the woman who helped him up, my mother.

Why did I choose a life as a doctor compassionate to animals? I am not completely sure. Was it because I preferred to treat the unprejudiced, silent species, known to respond with love to any kindness? Do I generally like animals more than humans? I like to think not.

There have been so many, Black and white and other colors of people, who helped me become the person I am today. Like Grace Hooks, a Black woman who graduated from Cornell University in 1930. Hearing her stories of resiliency in the face of racism and discrimination while she attended college and visited her mother in Alabama taught me patience, humility, and generosity. Carl Osborne, my PhD adviser, who was white, cared for me as if I were one of his sons. In him, I found the unconditional love and guidance my father was incapable of providing. My teachers who encouraged me and my clients who appreciated my compassion kept me going. I did not do this alone.

And then there were those who slowed me down. I usually worked late. Caring for my patients and my students demanded that of me. In September 2015, I looked up at the clock after reading a chapter on kidney failure and was stunned that it was almost 8:00 p.m. I had promised to be home by 7:00 p.m. I gathered up my two dogs, who come to work with me every day, and rushed to the car. The speed limit on campus was twenty miles per hour. I was going faster. When I turned onto Larpenteur Avenue, flashing lights from behind ordered me to stop. I pulled over and the police car parked behind me. The officer said that I was going thirty-eight miles per hour. He wanted to see my license. My dogs in the front seat barked incessantly at him. I apologized and explained that they were alarmed by an unfamiliar person standing so close. Then I explained that my wallet with my license was in my backpack, and it was on the floor in front of the passenger seat. I asked if it was okay for me to get it. Most of my Black friends would understand why I was so cautious. I didn't want the policeman to get nervous, thinking that I was reaching for a gun. To make matters worse, my dogs kept barking. I handed the officer my license. He stepped back behind the car and the dogs quieted down. After a few minutes, he came back to the driver side window and handed my license back to me. He gave me a warning and not a speeding ticket and sent me on my way. I was relieved. Nine months later, I was horrified as I watched the evening news. That same cop *during a routine traffic stop* had just shot and killed Philando Castile, *a young Black man, on the same street, just blocks from where he stopped me for a routine traffic stop. That could have been me.*

On my way through life, I have learned much. Being a Black man, there are things I have had to accept: feeling unsafe and afraid to speak up, being unheard and considered dispensable, having your accomplishments dismissed as affirmative action, and living with the loneliness of being the only one in the department, the classroom, the clinic, and my college. But I was lucky. I did not become a statistic even though my past was fertilizer for failure.

It is my hope that after reading my memoir, you will come away not with a sense of sorrow for the misfortunes I endured but with a sense of resiliency for the courage to always lead with my heart. It is not the actions of others that defeat us but the sense of hopelessness that paralyzes us. I was nine years old when my mother died. I was devastated. I vowed never to trust or love anyone again. I thought that in isolation I would be safe. But a life without love is not a life worth living. It took me a long time to find that out. When I did, my life changed.

I survived because others loved me. And because I eventually let them. They showed me how to turn pain and sorrow into something bigger. They showed me that we can succeed, not in spite of a difficult past, but because of it.

PART I

MOTHER

1

NEW YEAR'S EVE

Outside, the air was cold enough to crystallize water into lace, but the ground was too warm to let it last, at least not while the sun was still up. Inside our house, I was drawn to the window by the falling snow. I stood close, amazed as each snowflake drifted past, floated to the ground, and melted, silent in its own death. That was how my mother would have had it, or so she tried. She remained quiet and withdrawn until the very end.

It started late in the afternoon on New Year's Eve in 1966. My mother and my father began screaming at each other. I was not sure what ignited their falling-out this time. The reasons were often inconsequential to the real problems: my mother's depression, our lack of money, and their habitual drinking. At the peak of their shouting match, my father pulled his wedding ring from his finger, cocked his arm over his head, and prepared to throw it at her.

My mother stopped bickering and began apologizing and then crying. My father hesitated. He didn't throw the ring, but he didn't put it back on his finger. Instead, he closed his hand, making a tight fist around it. He ran to the basement. As quickly as he scooted off, he returned, carrying a sledgehammer. With my mother watching, he placed his wedding ring on top of the dresser and stood the ring on its edge. I heard him grimace as he brought down the sledgehammer. It hit the ring, making a loud thud, flattening the gold band and obliterating the opening where his finger once fit. He picked up the mutilated symbol of their marriage and this time, with all of his ferocity, threw it at her. But if that were not enough, as the ring hurtled through the air, he screamed, "Get out of my life!"

The ring hit my mother square across the chest and fell to the bed without making a sound. For a brief moment, silence filled the house as we all held our breath. Then my father's footsteps thundered past me as he stormed out of the bedroom and out of the house, leaving the front door wide open as he left. The wind rushed in and filled me with a chill that I still remember. I closed the door and returned to check on my mother.

She looked down at the flattened metal object that was once my father's wedding ring. She stopped sobbing. She wiped the tears from her face and the saliva from her lips. She sat up, got out of bed, and walked to the back of the house and into the kitchen. She reached under the cabinet, pulled out a dark plastic bottle, and from it poured a green liquid into a small glass. She stared at the glass. Then with both hands, she lifted it to her mouth and drank its contents. Her lips pursed and her eyes closed. When she opened her eyes, I was standing in front of her. She put the glass down and stepped toward me. She reached down and passed her hand through my hair. Her hand stopped when it reached the back of my head. Then she exhaled a stuttering whimper.

I wanted to comfort her. I wanted her to reach out and pull me in close. When she didn't, I looked up. She slowly shook her head from side to side, but only once. Without saying a word, she slid her hand down the back of my neck and over my right shoulder. Then, she let go of me. She turned around, slowly walked back to the bedroom, and retreated under the bed covers. As she lifted the blankets to get in bed, I heard my father's wedding ring clink as it fell to the floor.

The night was quiet; I fell asleep in my bed. When I woke the next morning, my father had returned and my mother started vomiting. At first, the sound was muffled. As if she did not want anyone to hear.

This was not the first time that silence would be her strength. Neither was it the first time that she threatened suicide. Once, she shoved pills in her mouth and ran out the back door. She knew that we were watching. She knew that we would go after her. And we did. We chased her and brought her back screaming while resisting our help.

That time, my father forced her to drink milk to coat her stomach. He pinched her nose. He pushed his fingers into the back of her throat, forcing her to choke and gag. He did it again and again until the contents of her stomach rose up into the back of her throat and white foam spewed from her mouth and nose, flooding the floor beneath her and at the same time spraying a white mist over me. Then she sobbed while promising never to do that again. But she did do it again. Over and over. So much so that her threats became less credible. But this time was different. She was weak. She did not have the strength to run. She did not have the strength to vomit, but she could not stop it. The vomiting continued as if something inside her were forcing itself up against her will, her body emptying everything from her abdomen through her mouth.

I heard liquid hit the floor. There was a pause. Then I heard *splat* as liquid hit the floor again. After a few more, there was nothing left but moaning and retching, so much so that my father worried and feared the worst. He let go of his anger from the night before and rushed to her side. He pleaded with her to know what it was this time. My mother answered by closing her mouth, turning away, and drawing in at the middle. She moaned in pain, but without uttering a single recognizable word. My father leaned into her again, put his mouth close to her ear, and begged, "Tell me what is wrong."

Again, she remained silent. Like pity drawing out sorrow, her silence lured my father in deeper, and she knew it. But she could not hold her position long. Against her will and the need to vomit, her body unraveled as she opened her mouth wide, extended her neck, and spewed out the final contents of her stomach.

I saw it all. I had been there from the beginning. The night before, I watched her fill the glass with green liquid. I watched her drink it. Someone besides my mother and me needed to know what she had done to herself. I could have stood up and headed for their bedroom door, tearing a hole in her silence wide enough to walk through and carry her with me. But I didn't. I could have, but I didn't. I remained by her side and said nothing. I assumed she wanted me not to.

It did not matter. My father had enough. He called my brother to get her coat. He leaned down over her in bed. He took her left arm and wrapped it around the back of his neck. He heaved her up. As her body uncoiled from the weight of her legs pulling her down, she grimaced a horrifying wail, revealing to us that her pain was real, so much so that she barely let her feet touch the floor. Then my father lifted her legs and carried her out to the car.

I watched through the window as they left. My brother opened the passenger door. My father lowered my mother into the back seat. My brother got in the car on the other side. With my hands pressed firmly against the glass, I could not turn away. The engine started. Exhaust spewed out the back. The car heaved slightly as my father engaged the clutch. Then the car sped away from the curve and disappeared down the street and into the darkness.

I remained fixed to the window. The street was covered in a blanket of white snow except for the bare square that was beneath our parked car. I stared at that space for a long time. I did not move until the falling snow filled the hole, obliterating the place where our car once stood.

I was not aware of the extent of my mother's desire to hurt herself until I walked into their bedroom. Once I did, I could tell from the vomit on the pillow, and the bed covers and sheets, and the floor, and the wall, that it had gone on too long. I shook my head and closed my eyes. I left their bedroom for my bed. I pulled the covers over my head. I tried to sleep but couldn't. My mind raced through all the possibilities. How long would she need to stay in the hospital? Was she coming back? I worried about what my life would look like without my mother. I wondered who would take care of me if she did not survive.

2

1957

I was born on September 15, 1957, in Michael Reese Hospital on Chicago's South Side. My mother kept records in a tan photo album with the words *Our Baby* on the cover. I remembered her telling me that I was a happy baby.

I still have that photo album. It is more than fifty years old. When I open it, the spine cracks and groans. It smells old and musty. The cellophane pockets holding the photographs have yellowed and splintered. On the inside cover, it's written that I was born at three o'clock in the afternoon and weighed seven and a half pounds. On the bottom of the page is a place for the signatures of my mother and my father, the doctor, and the nurse, but all the lines are blank. As I open the album, several pictures slip out of their jackets and fall into my lap. Some have dark edges and frayed corners as if they had been handled often. Some are well preserved without a crease or crack. My mother was right. In these pictures, I am smiling. My toothless, chubby-cheeked grin repeats itself in one picture after another.

I was six years old when my mother first showed me the album. It was a hot summer evening. We were home alone. My older brother was outside horsing around with friends. My father was working a second shift at the cereal plant where he made Wheaties. She called me into the living room and patted the empty spot next to her on the couch. I eagerly flopped down. The sides of my legs rubbed against hers.

She reached overhead and turned on the light behind us, opened the album, and asked, "Do you know who that is in the picture?"

I said, "It's me," while tapping my fingers to my chest.

She smiled in agreement and leaned back. I leaned back into her. She turned more pages and passed more photographs. I watched her smile and remember an earlier time. Then she turned to face me and said, "Your father and I worried over you from the first day you were born."

Worry over me? Why, I thought. You said that I was a happy baby.

"When you were two days old, your father came to the hospital to bring us home."

At the time of my birth, our home was a prewar, three-flat, brick apartment building. It was built at a time when labor was cheap and craftsmanship was prized. A time when front stoops and front stairs were cut from stone. A time when ceilings were tall, heat traveled through pipes in the floor to radiators perched against interior walls, and walls were thick and impenetrable. We lived on the first floor in a two-bedroom apartment with a large living room and a small kitchen.

"After parking the car, your father rushed to the other side and opened the passenger door. I cradled you in one arm and used my other arm to lift myself up from the seat. Your father helped. Once up, he leaned into me. Our foreheads lightly touched before we rested into each other. We both smiled and whispered how perfectly you would fit into the family, how you would sleep between us in our bed, and how your tiny fingers would rest in the gentle grasp of your older brother's reach.

"As we walked up the curb to the stoop of our apartment building, your father was cautious. There were only three steps to the top of our stoop. On the first step, he braced his arms below you, in case I dropped you. You were not my first child. He knew that I knew how to carry a baby. Then he relaxed and instead fixed his gaze on you, your smooth brown skin and your wispy hair swirled into waves on the top of your head. He noticed that you had his nose and his tall forehead. You began to smile. We felt nothing but joy. However, before reaching the top of our stoop, your father stopped in midstep. I was behind and almost collided into him. The newspaper, usually tightly rolled and fastened with a red rubber band, instead lay open. Splayed across the front page was a picture of a Black teenage girl surrounded by an angry white mob. Your father looked up at me. I had not seen the newspaper, but was good at reading his face. I knew that something was wrong. I followed his line of sight and saw the picture that worried him. In an instant, seeing that picture unfolded a memory all too familiar to us. Instead of finishing the short climb up and into the apartment, we stopped and sat on the wide stone railing of the stoop of our apartment building.

"You were asleep in my arms, which is where we needed you to stay. Only then did your father reach down and pick up the newspaper and take a closer look.

"I leaned into him, so much so that he tilted the newspaper in my direction. Then we read the caption together, *white students shout insults at Elizabeth Eckford, a fourteen-year-old negro as she marches down a line of guardsmen who block the entrance to Little Rock school.* In the photograph, Elizabeth Eckford was impeccably dressed in a white, starched, short-sleeve blouse and light-colored cotton skirt. She wore large sunglasses, perhaps hiding the fear on her face from the crowd collecting around her. Her school notebook and pencil pouch secured in her left arm and brought close to her chest not only contained what she needed for school but gave her something to hold on to, because in those unpleasant predicaments— you always need something to hold on to. She was moving cautiously away from the crowd, even though she had, like every other student, the right to be there. She knew to tell herself to not look at them, to just keep walking and whatever you do—don't cry. Don't let them see you cry. She did not cry, but it was obvious from the crease in her brow, and her sucked-in lower lip, that somewhere, deep inside, endless tears flowed.

"The photographer was lucky. In a single frame, he captured not only the reticence of Elizabeth Eckford but the intense hatred in Hazel Bryan, the white teenager swiftly approaching from behind. She was perhaps the same age and dressed respectfully in a starched one-piece solid pastel dress with a cloth belt fastened close around her waist that formed a tight knot in the front. Her dark hair puffed up on her head before swooping back and stopping at her neck. Her lips parted wide and pulled tightly across her face, baring teeth like a snarling dog. Hazel did not wear sunglasses. She did not hide her dark beady eyes. She didn't have to. By the rush of her step and the sway of her shoulders, she knew that the crowd carried her forward. She knew that she was not alone. She also knew that she was on a collision course with Elizabeth Eckford.

"The caption did not say what Hazel was shouting at Elizabeth, but you knew from the shape of her mouth and the extension of her head, and the prominent veins in her neck. You knew from the color of her white skin, and the Ozark Mountains in the distance, and the discourse of the time."

*

"Crinkling the newspaper in his hand, your father looked down at that picture again—this time recalling the civil rights rally where he and I met. Like Elizabeth Eckford, he carefully avoided the white mob collecting behind him. He did not want to accept, and did not want them to know, the fear collecting inside him. And so, he too would keep moving forward. And by doing so, he did not see the young man off to his left finish his beer. He did not see him take the empty bottle and hold it firmly around its neck. He did not see the young man swing the beer bottle over his head ratcheting up momentum, kick his leg out and stomp it down, uncoiling his body while hurling the bottle in the air on a trajectory toward the crowd.

"Your father did not know that all the while, through the windup, the release, and the exuberant grunt, that the young man would keep his eyes on him because the young man knew that one white face in the crowd was more of a threat to his terrorizing mission than a sea of all Black ones. When the bottle landed on mark, hitting its intended target, your father would fall to the ground and not see anything for what seemed like hours. And when he fell to the ground he would not hear the young man hatefully shout, *Nigger lover.* What your father would remember was the beautiful brown-skinned woman who helped him up from the pavement."

My mother brought her face closer to mine, confirming what I already knew. We both chuckled.

"While sitting on the front stoop, your father looked up from the newspaper and then looked down at you. You were still asleep. However, for a brief moment, his enthusiasm for bringing you home drained from his face and the air from his lungs filled his cheeks with worry, so much so that he pondered if the world would create a safe place for you or teach you to hate. When his expression changed to worry, I held you tighter as if to protect you. But I didn't stay there long. I knew that I couldn't protect you. Instead, I believed that you would be safe. That the world would change. That it was not fear you needed, but love."

*

For as far back as I can remember, my mother always told me stories like this. She would tell me the stories of the warriors of history, Black and white and all the shades in between. She'd tell me the story of her father going to college at a time when Black men were lynched for just thinking of an education. She'd tell me these stories as if she were preparing me for a world of contradictions and injustices. She'd tell me these stories as if I had the wisdom of an old man, but at the time, I was a little boy. After telling me these stories, she'd hug me. She'd hold me so tight that I could hardly breathe. And then she did what she said she had to. She layered me in love: unconditional, unfaltering, persistent love. She knew that she had to fill me with so much love that no matter what gets taken away, there would always be enough left to carry me through the most difficult times. And while my mother and my father were conjuring up all the defenses for protecting me from the uncontrollable inequities on the outside, what none of us knew at the time was that it would be the misunderstandings, the abuse, and the unrecognized mental illness on the inside of our family that would be our biggest challenge to overcome.

3

DAD

The summer of 1961 was unbearably hot. The warm air lapped up the moisture rising off Lake Michigan, and the mugginess hung there for weeks, permeating my clothes and making my skin slippery. I was almost four years old and was miserable because there was nothing that I could do to escape it. Air conditioning was a rarity, and our apartment was no exception. Lake Michigan was less than a mile away, but without supervision, I was not permitted near the water. What I cherished about that summer was how every weekend we escaped the heat by going to the drive-in movie. Saturday nights as the sun began its arc downward on the west, tall shadows of the apartment buildings on my block stretched across the road. My brother and I would pile into the back seat of our car. My mother sat up front with my father as he drove from our apartment building in the Hyde Park neighborhood near the University of Chicago. We arrived before dusk and parked in the center near the front of the big movie screen. My mom packed sandwiches and soda, but sometimes we were lucky enough to have fried chicken and potato salad. We had an evening picnic in the car as the temperature dropped with the setting sun.

We lifted the clunky movie speaker from the post outside the car. It was a gray metal box the size of a thick novel. Multiple slats on the front allowed the sound to come out of the speakers. A wide hook on the back secured it to the window. After attaching the speaker, we rolled up the window to keep it in place.

When the movie started, the large screen cast a white glow, blanching the night sky with a white beam. My father leaned into my mother. He placed his arm over her shoulder. They moved closer together, giving me an unobstructed view of the movie from the back seat. But after eating so much food, it was not long before the sounds of the summer night crickets outside lulled me to sleep.

I would not wake up until after the drive back home. My father parked the car outside our apartment.

We had a ritual. I knew that if I pretended to be asleep, my father would carry me in and put me to bed. I remained perfectly still and patiently waited.

My father cuts the engine. He looks over his shoulder and watches me in the back seat. I keep my eyes closed and do not move.

He whispers to my mother and brother, "Be quiet, don't move, I'll take him in." He slowly opens the driver's side and quietly steps out. He remembers not to let the car door slam closed on its own. Instead, he gently leans the door against its latch. Using the weight of his hip, he gives it a soft nudge. The latch clicks and the door closes with barely a sound.

He quietly walks around to the back of the car. From inside the car, my mother lifts the latch and unlocks the passenger door. The door next to me opens. He reaches below me to take hold of any part that might dangle out. But nothing dangles out. He scoops me up as if he were holding me for the first time. I can't help but smile. I stretch slightly and curl up against his chest. I fit perfectly into the cradle that he creates out of his bowed arms and cupped torso. Tilting me toward him, he holds me closer. I hear his heart beating through his shirt. I feel as if I were a part of him, as if he could tell me everything on his mind without a word passing between us. I feel as if there were no one else but us. At that moment, my lips part and I murmur a sigh of pure gratification. Only then does he nod, giving my mother and my brother permission to exit the car, but not before he utters a low long *shhhhhhhh,* reminding them to move slowly and close the car doors quietly.

With me in his arms, he turns in the direction of our apartment and walks over the grass to avoid the hard sidewalk. When he tiptoes up the stairs, I feel only the ascent and not the break at each step.

He carries me down the long hallway to the bedroom that I share with my brother. My mother knows not to turn on the light; the moonlight glimmering through the window is all the illumination we need. She steps in front of my father and folds back the bed covers. He places me in the top bunk on my back. He unlaces my shoes and gently slides them off. He pauses and looks down at me. He releases the snap on the waist of my pants. He gently tugs the right cuff and then the left, and then right, and then the left until my legs let go of my pants. He folds them over the footboard of the bed. He unbuttons my shirt and lifts it, gently slipping the sleeves from my right arm, across my back,

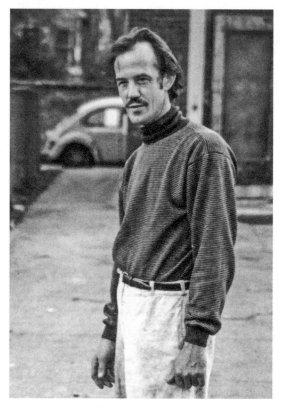

*My father in the backyard of our
Hyde Park–Kenwood home in 1979.*

and finally freeing my left arm. He leaves my undershirt, underwear, and socks on. He gently tilts me up on my right side. As I peer through tiny eye slits, he looks deep into my face before lowering me back in place. He lifts the covers, brings them forward, and lets them slowly fall over my body, leaving my head and shoulders exposed.

He rests his hand across my shoulder and chest so gently that I feel only the warmth of his palm. He stands there, watching me slowly breathe in and out. I hear his breathing. With each exhalation, I try to match his. A slow deep inhale, a slight pause, and a gentle release as his breath swirls over my head. Then I feel his entire body let go. The weight of his arm on my shoulder lets me know how much he loves me. I want to reach up and hold him, but I do not want to let him know that I am not asleep. He stretches out his thumb and gently strokes the hair on the back of my head. He gently opens and closes his hand, caressing my shoulder. An immense tenderness passes between us. I do not know how to explain it, but I feel completely safe and loved. I do not know how long he stays because I drift into sleep, deep and carefree sleep, as his tenderness imprints my consciousness with these images that stay with me forever.

As I look back, these are the images that kept me tethered to home, even later, when home became the place that frightened me most. These are the memories that bonded me to my father even years later as he pushed me away. And when he became old and frail, these are the images that drew me back to him.

4

FRIDAYS

On Friday nights, my father read the week's mail at the kitchen table over dinner. Our typical meal was meatloaf and mashed potatoes or chicken and dumplings. "Comfort food for the heart," my mother called it. Nothing too spicy, nothing too hot, and something that we all enjoyed. With our bellies full and our plates clean, my brother and I brought our empty dishes to the sink. My mother washed them and placed them on the rack to dry. My father, still in his work clothes and still eating slowly, made his way through the mail. Wearing white slacks and a white work shirt, he looked more like the milkman than a factory worker. His formidable dark-brown steel toe shoes with scuff marks and scratches told me otherwise.

He sat at the table with both feet flat on the floor and the light pouring over his shoulder. Going through the mail was his quiet time. My mother in her bare feet and tight-fitting blue jeans put her hand on his shoulder before ushering his plate to the sink with the other dirty dishes. He did not look up. She came back, sat down next to him, and with the back of her hand lightly stroked his cheek. He continued reading. She got up and walked into the living room and I followed her.

She stood in front of the console rhythmically tapping the top with her fingers. Off to the side was our record collection. She thumbed through the stack and set one to the side. I crawled up into a large comfortable chair, sat back against the cushion, and watched. She slid open the cover on the console that hid our record player. Carefully she removed the record from its jacket, held it up to the light, and selected the side she wanted to hear. She lowered the record into the console, placing it over the spindle in the center of the turntable. I heard a click of a knob, and the turntable started. She lifted the tonearm and placed the needle on the edge of the record. Crackling static exited the speakers before the needle made its way into the first song. And when it did, out poured a syncopated Latin beat with bongo drums and trumpets. The volume was low, but my mother's energy was ramping up. Her body began to sway with the beat as she shifted her weight from one foot onto the other. She added in her hips. When her right leg bent at the knee, her right shoulder dipped in front, and her left hip went out to the side. With each movement, her toes arched, digging into the rug. She closed her eyes and gently rocked from side to side. When the first song ended, her tongue arched over her upper lip as if she had just tasted the most delicious chocolate. She opened her eyes, turned her head, and looked into the kitchen. My father, still inspecting the week's mail, had hardly budged.

The next song started with a faster beat. She turned the volume up. Her feet began to move. Three steps forward and two quick steps in place. Then three steps backward. At the time, I didn't know it, but she was dancing the mambo or the cha-cha. She stepped hard, leaving impressions in the rug as she moved across the living room floor. When she stepped sideways, her arms stylishly moved in unison with her feet. She danced in my direction, luring me to join her. As she came closer, my eyes widened. On the next beat, she made a 180-degree turn and danced backward while still moving toward me. As she approached, I arched my back deep into the cushion of the chair. Three beats later, she turned again, this time moving away from me, and kept dancing by herself. In the middle of the song, her eyes caught mine and she quickly advanced toward me again. As she approached, she held both hands out with her palms up, inviting me to join her. I scooched to the edge of the chair. She came closer. I felt the beat and knew exactly when to launch. I reached out anticipating our connection, but before we touched, my father stepped between us. I had not seen him get up from the table. I had not heard him take off his clunky work shoes. He stood between us in his stocking feet.

He laid his hands in hers, looked into her eyes, and moved in close. Then the next song started. My mother's hips swayed seductively. She and my father held on to each other and crisscrossed the floor, bending their bodies to the syncopated beat.

When I was older, my aunt on my mother's side told me that my mother grew up in a household of sisters who danced. "There were six of us, and your uncle Buddy," she said. "On weekends after the adults sat down for a game of gin rummy or bid whist, we girls headed for the front porch. We turned up the radio and dialed in the soul stations, WGES or WJJD, or took a stack of records to spin on the record player. Take the A Train, Slippin' and Slidin', Let the Good Times Roll, and Cupid's Boogie filled the house with strong Afro-Latin beats that were too irresistible to sit. You had to get up and move," my aunt laughed out loud. "Us girls gathered together swinging our hips and moving our arms to the thumping backbeat. The older ones taught the younger ones to do the swing, the jitterbug, the cha-cha-cha, and the twist. The younger ones goofily flopped around moving their hands wildly as if they just touched a hot stove. Boy, you should have seen your aunt Shirley; she had the smooth seductive movements of a leopard."

I responded by saying, "I can see it today in the way Aunt Shirley walks. With her long legs and slim hips, she glides down the sidewalks."

Watching my mother and my father do the mambo and cha-cha, I was four years old going on five, but I wanted to dance like the adults. I watched my parents move across the floor with electrifying precision. My shoulders swayed with theirs, but my clumsy feet didn't know what to do. I slid out of the big chair and knelt on the floor for a closer look. Seeing me on the floor, Lightning, our black cocker spaniel, came over, sat close, and leaned into me. We were both mesmerized by the synchronization of my parents' dance movements. When my mother stepped forward to the beat, my father, in unison, stepped backward. When side by side, they moved left and then right with identical footwork. Just when I thought that it could not get any better, my father twirled my mother in place; when she stopped, he twirled in place next to her, all while holding her hand and holding on to the beat. Watching them shuffle across the carpet while they laughed and giggled, and stuck their tongues out at each other, made me roar with excitement.

When the last song ended, the turntable kept spinning. A low crackling sound poured out of the speakers, waiting for someone to lift the tonearm and turn off the motor. The sound of my mother's and my father's breathing filled the room too. Their chests rose and lowered in unison. Their shiny faces glowed with perspiration and intent. They approached each other slowly. She came in close, turned around, leaned her back into his chest, and rested the back of her head on his shoulder. My father stepped forward catching her and wrapped one arm around her waist. He slid his hand under the front of her sweater and splayed his hand against her belly, gently passing his fingers over her smooth skin while dipping his little finger into her navel. She leaned in, closing any space between them, this time tilting her face into the angle formed where his neck and shoulder met.

Lightning wanted the same show of affection. He leaned deeper into my side, so much so that he flopped to the floor. As he rested on his side, he pressed against my leg and arched his back, exposing his belly. I reached down and swirled my fingers through his long curly fur. I flattened my hand, spreading it across his abdomen, and gently massaged his belly, crisscrossing over his navel. He closed his eyes and gave his body another full stretch. That was when I heard a faint coo fall from his half-opened mouth as he exhaled.

When I got out of bed the next morning, my father was at the kitchen table, finishing the job of opening the mail. My mother didn't get out of bed until later. Seeing us at the table, she sat close to my father, lightly kissed his cheek, and joined us for breakfast.

5

LAKU NOĆ

I knew little about my family on my father's side. What I did know I learned from conversations I overheard between my mother and my father, and the times I visited Grandma Lulich when I was a child. My father's parents emigrated from eastern Europe. At that time, it was Yugoslavia, but today it is Croatia. They immigrated to America in the 1920s. They came because of economic hardship and poverty, to make a better living in America because it was impossible to do so in their homeland. When they arrived, Grandpa Lulich found work in the steel mills of Chicago. Grandma Lulich was a secretary in a small office and managed the books.

I never met Grandpa Lulich. He died several months before I was born. My mother hated him. She had her reasons. "Grandpa Lulich held on to old beliefs and old ways," she said. "He could not look beyond the brown color of my skin and the texture of my hair to see the person I am on the inside and accept the woman his son loved and married. Grandpa Lulich told your father to not bring that *crnackog* (negro) woman in his house ever again."

In the 1950s, when my mother and father got married, the term *Negro* was popular for members of the African American race. I trust that this is how Grandpa Lulich said it. But I was not there. When my mother tells the story, she uses the word *negro* and not the word *nigger*.

My mother added, "For all the difficulties that Grandpa Lulich had to overcome to immigrate to America, to find work, and to make a home here, why couldn't he find the compassion and empathy for others who had gone through similar struggles? Why did it take his impending death to see differently?"

At the age of sixty-nine, three years after my parents' marriage, Grandpa Lulich developed rapidly progressing leukemia. With only months to live, he abandoned his bigotry and opened his heart. He sought reconciliation and begged for forgiveness.

For my father, a simple apology was all that was needed. My father would visit him often after his diagnosis. My mother, on the other hand, held on to her animosity and stayed at home. My older brother, Gary, who was only two at the time, would stay home with her.

As Grandpa Lulich became sicker and more aware of his frailty, he sought strength and purpose in his life by correcting his mistakes. He knew that my mother was very angry and hurt for the things he said in the past. If he could have, he would have left the hospital and asked for her forgiveness in person, but he was too sick to leave the hospital. Since my mother would not come to him, he begged my father to ask her if she would at least allow him to see his grandson, Gary. During my father's next visit, Gary came with him, but my mother stayed home.

"Gary, this is your grandpa," my father said as he introduced the two to each other. Grandpa Lulich smiled and waved for Gary to come closer. As Gary came closer, Grandpa Lulich nodded and, in a weak voice, said, "I am happy to meet you." Feeling at ease with a man he had never seen before, Gary leaned in closer. My father hoisted Gary up and sat him on the edge of the hospital bed. Grandpa Lulich affectionately placed his hand around Gary's waist to support him and with the back of his other hand lightly stroked Gary's face. Grandpa Lulich looked up at my father and said, "He looks just like you, doesn't he?"

When Gary came home, he told my mother what a great time he had. He told her that Grandpa Lulich was gentle and kind. He told my mother that Grandpa Lulich kept saying that he was sorry, but Gary didn't know what for. Then Gary told my mother that Grandpa Lulich wanted to see her too. After hearing these things, my mother softened. She was never good at keeping a grudge for long. From then on, they would visit Grandpa Lulich in the hospital as a family. He was appreciative of their company.

At the time of Grandpa Lulich's death, my mother would have been six months pregnant with me and showing it. At the end of his life, I imagined the relationship between Grandpa Lulich and my mother grew exponentially, for they had little time left and a lot of catching up to do, and a lot of forgiveness to consider between them both. I imagined that during one of those final visits, Grandpa Lulich gently placed his hand over my mother's pregnant belly and had a wish for me. Maybe for good health and long life. Or maybe he hoped that my mother would speak kindly of him after he passed, when I was old enough to understand who he was.

She kept that promise. She told me the truth about Grandpa Lulich. Her words could have been terse and unrelenting. Instead, she spoke kindly of him with much empathy. She reminded me that times were different then and that Grandpa Lulich was treated badly because of his position in life in Croatia. She would tell me that being an immigrant and trying to fit in here was difficult for him. She would tell me that sometimes people are too proud of who they have become to remember where they started. In the end, she would tell me that he was a kind man.

*

Unlike Grandpa Lulich, Grandma Lulich was a woman of few words. She was not very demonstrative with her affection, but she was overflowing with her nurturing.

When my parents dropped me off at her house, Grandma Lulich was happy to see me. She'd crouch down and smile so close to my face, I could smell the coffee on her breath, but she was not very cuddly. She did not pinch my cheeks or give me big warm hugs. After opening the door and ushering me inside, she would reach for her floral apron from the back of her easy chair, slip it over her head, and tie the loose straps around her waist. Then she'd reach for my hands and lead me down the long hallway to the kitchen. I eagerly followed. When we reached the kitchen, she'd pull a chair out from under the kitchen table, point to it, and in her Serbo-Croatian accent, tell me to sit.

It sounded like she was saying *seat,* the noun, which I would have called a chair, instead of *sit,* the verb.

"Okay Grandma, I seat," I said, making fun of her accent. She'd come in close, stand over me and purse her lips and nod her head before turning around and igniting a fire under a small pot of water on the kitchen stove. Grandma Lulich knew how to make only one dish, poached eggs. Whether it was breakfast, lunch, or dinner, it was always poached eggs. This visit would not be different. She opened the refrigerator and took out two eggs. After the water rigorously boiled, she'd move the pan off the heat to a cold burner on the stove and quickly crack the eggs, emptying their contents into the hot water. Then she'd cut a thick slice of bread from the loaf on the counter, spear the side of it with a fork, and lightly toast it over the open flame. With my toast came a glass of milk. After the eggs were poached, she'd scoop them from the hot water, plop them on the toast, and push the plate in my direction.

"Eat," she'd say, with her English clearer this time.

I pierced the eggs with my fork and orange yolk oozed out, soaking the toast. She'd sit across from me and tap her finger on the table near my plate, encouraging me to finish every bite. I imagined hard times in Croatia where food was scarce, and when you had it, you finished every morsel. I was not particularly fond of poached eggs. But I liked the attention she showed me while I was eating them.

When I was done, she'd slide my chair back from the kitchen table, take my hand in hers, and lead me to the bedroom.

"Naptime," she'd say. A dark mahogany, four-poster bed sat against the middle of the far wall of her small bedroom. A beige cotton bedspread with a large embroidered medallion in the center neatly covered the mattress and pillows. After taking off my shoes, she'd lift the covers and fold me under them. The sheets were sparkling white and a little stiff, as if they had dried outside on a clothesline in the sun. With me on my back and the covers up to my neck, she'd lean over and gently wipe the crumbs from my cheeks and lips. I'd feel her warm hands brush against my skin. That was about as affectionate as Grandma Lulich got.

"Go to sleep," she'd say. After she turned off the light, and while slowly closing the door, I'd hear her whisper, "Laku Noć."

The first time I heard those words, I could not make out what she was saying. For all I knew, she said I'm locking the door, or don't pee in the bed. But I recalled something familiar in her words. Quiet evenings when my father was particularly paternal and put me to bed, I would hear him say the same phrase. After turning off the bedroom light and before closing the door, he said, "Laku Noć." Other times, when he thought that I was asleep, he'd lean over me, kiss my forehead, and in my ear whisper, "Laku Noć." It didn't take me long to figure out what it meant. At my next visit, when Grandma Lulich turned off the bedroom light, peered her head around a half-closed door, and whispered, "Laku Noć, " I turned in her direction and whispered back into the darkness, "Good night, Grandma."

6

MOM

At night, when I couldn't sleep or was afraid to fall back to sleep because of the creatures in my closet, I'd climb out of bed, walk down the hallway, and stand at my parents' bedroom door. I didn't want to wake them but hoped they'd notice the worry on my face and the shifting of my feet. After watching them sleep with no inclination of waking, I'd lean in and whisper, "Mom?"

From out of the darkness, she'd whisper back, "Come on in, baby."

I would follow her voice and carefully advance until my feet met the edge of their bed. Then I'd reach down, and my hand would sink into the soft beige comforter my mother knitted. Beneath the comforter, I'd feel my father's feet. I was careful not to wake him.

I'd count three steps to the left: one, two, three. That would place me on the side of the bed where my mother slept. I'd bend down slightly and glide my fingers along the bottom edge of the covers, feeling for an opening. Finding one, I'd slowly lift the covers. My mother would reach out and gently gobble me up in her arms. Her body was warm. She'd lower me down next to her and pull me close. Only then would my breath stretch back into sleep.

I visited my parents' bedroom often, so much so that I could navigate the layout of their room in total darkness. Just inside the door on the wall was the light switch. I knew not to touch that switch for fear of waking them.

Against the same wall stood a low oak dresser with two rows of drawers. Whenever I hurt myself playing outside, my mother would sit me on top of that dresser. With my legs dangling over one side, she'd clear the tears from my eyes and wipe the dirt and blood from the scrapes on my hands and knees. She'd look up at me and, behind a smile, remind me to slow down and be more careful next time. I'd nod. Then she'd untie the laces on my shoes, slip the shoes from my feet, and we'd spend the rest of the afternoon in bed. My pain and foolishness quickly evaporated into thin air.

To the left of the dresser was a large closet with sliding doors. I'd lean in with all my weight. The doors would slowly open. I'd climb inside, lie on the floor, and look up at the kaleidoscope of colors and textures of my mother's clothes suspended on their hangers above me.

My mom was a consummate tailor. She sat for hours at her sewing machine, stitching together the most beautiful clothes.

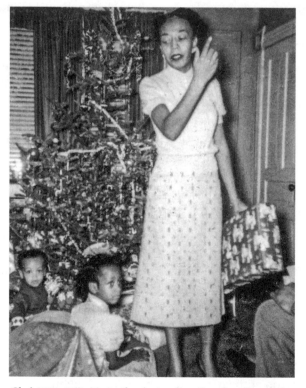

Christmas 1959. My mother is standing. I am kneeling under the tree on the left, and my aunt Tanya is between us.

A trip to the fabric store made her giddy and joyful. As she entered, her eyes would light up. She'd find inspiration walking the aisles. With her fingers lightly passing over each sample, she'd imagine the finished product: a pleated skirt, a matador's jacket with no buttons, a blouse with a French cuff, no, a two-button mitered cuff, and a Peter Pan collar. She had a fondness for bold patterns with meandering lines. Anything pink made her smile.

We'd enter the house with bundles of fabric. She'd dump everything out on the dining room table. Without a pattern, she would measure, cut, and sew sumptuous pieces into beautiful outfits. When they were near completion, she'd fit the clothes over her dress form. It was jarring for me to see this headless, armless, legless mannequin perched on its base, wearing my mother's clothes. The first time she brought the mannequin home, I tentatively walked up to it and tapped it with my finger. I wanted to know if it was alive. Spongy fabric covered hard plastic underneath. It was not alive, but in the dark, it frightened me. I had nightmares that even without a head, it watched my every move.

When she finished her creations, she took them off the dress form and hung them in her closet. Her clothes were arranged by season, starting with her dark-brown wool coat and matching tweed pants. When it snowed, I'd watch her stuff the cuffs of those pants into her boots to keep her feet dry. Watching her, I did the same with my pants. I loved feeling her winter clothes. They were thick and textured. After a few more pairs of pants and another coat, the colors shifted from browns to lively shades of green and blue. Full-skirted swing dresses in simple solids signaled warmer weather and longer days. Then came the summer collection, dresses with short sleeves and open backs. The fabrics were lighter, the lapels narrower, and the dresses shorter. A gray form-fitting pencil dress with a tailored white collar and white cuffs on long sleeves transitioned her wardrobe into the fall. This shin-length creation provided an air of elegance, with its row of black buttons from the hem to the heart. It was her fall clothing that showcased her amazing talents.

I am not sure what got my mother sewing. I assumed that she learned it from her parents or in high school. But a stroll down Michigan Avenue with her proved that sewing was not only a joy but also a necessity.

Midmorning, we hopped on a commuter bus to downtown. After crossing the bridge above the Chicago River, we strolled up Michigan Avenue. North of downtown, Michigan Avenue was called the Magnificent Mile. It was known for its luxury shops that catered to Chicago's most affluent residents.

My mother loved window-shopping the Mile. Her ideas spawned from seeing what the mannequins were wearing. At first, nothing caught her eye. But when we detoured down a side street, she immediately stopped. In the window was the most beautiful dress she had ever seen, made of beige linen with over a thousand stitches of embroidery over the top and halfway down its short sleeves. Embroidered acanthus leaves and other Victorian scrolls imparted a subtle elegance to the dress. The color of the stitching flawlessly matched the color of the cloth, creating an embossing that would have been missed by any ordinary onlooker, but not my mother. She moved in closer and peered in the window, examining the dress's construction and admiring the artistry.

Grabbing my hand, she dragged me behind her, and we rushed into the shop. When she saw the back of the dress, her mouth dropped. The embroidery on the front continued over the shoulders, down the back, and gradually narrowed until it tapered to a single thread in the middle. I thought that my mother was going to scream in delight, but she maintained her decorum and contained her enthusiasm.

The sales clerk walked toward us and, with a slight lift of her head, asked, "Can I help you?"

My mother's eyes lit up like a beacon. She turned to the sales clerk and, in her most polite voice, said, "I would like to try this one on."

The woman didn't respond right away. Instead, she straightened her back, looked up into my mother's face, and in her most authoritative voice said, "Sorry, we do not have that dress in your size."

How would she know my mother's size?

My mother's eyes narrowed. It was obvious that the sales clerk assumed that my mother was not white enough or not rich enough to try on that dress.

My mother's decorum shifted. She raised an outstretched arm, pushing her open palm within inches of the woman's nose. My mother was not a traffic cop, but the way she positioned herself would have immediately halted all the cars on Michigan Avenue. The sales clerk shut up and stepped back.

Without saying a word, my mother turned around and grabbed my hand so tightly it hurt. She didn't let go until we were out of that shop and back on Michigan Avenue. With my hand free, I shook it to force the blood back into my fingers.

We got back on the bus and went home. Once inside, my mother made a beeline for her sewing machine. I thought that she was going to stitch together the dress of her dreams, the beige linen with acanthus leaves embroidered over the shoulders and sleeves. To my surprise, she never made that dress, but every dress she crafted after our encounter with that sales clerk was a stunning masterpiece that fitted my mother perfectly.

7

MOVING

In the fall of 1962, I turned five years old, and it was as if the world flipped on its side. We packed up our belongings and left the stately gray-stone apartment building with its tall ceilings and long hallways. We left the old man who operated the small corner drugstore across the street. Inside his shop, the walls were dark wood panels. From a bronzed tin ceiling hung several old schoolhouse lights with wide milk-glass shades. In the center hung a fan with slowly rotating blades that provided a gentle breeze. In the corner nestled a soda fountain with seats and a bench. He would sit my brother and me at the counter and feed us Lifesavers candy and cream sodas. He talked about how the war and the persecution of Jews forced him to leave his country and move to the United States. Not fully understanding what he was trying to convey, we listened and enjoyed his generosity, and now we were moving.

When we moved, we left the comfort of big open spaces, Lake Michigan, the Museum of Science and Industry, and the mile-long Midway Park alongside the University of Chicago. Wide-open spaces made me feel secure. I could look up and see the stars. Or look out across the lake and see the horizon and the rising sun. Wide-open spaces muffled the nervous noise of the city that sometimes frightened me.

We moved because my father wanted to own his home instead of paying rent. He saved his earnings, worked extra shifts at his factory job, and purchased our first house. It was not a move up. Our new home was an old dark-brown, wood-frame duplex that sat in the middle of the sixty-ninth block of Cornell Avenue. The back porch was falling down. The front porch slanted toward the front yard. The first time I climbed up the front stairs, the old wood railing leading up to the porch jabbed a sliver into my hand. Nevertheless, it was our home instead of paying rent.

As soon as we settled in, everything fell apart, not the house, but our lives. After the move, for the first time, I saw my father punch my mother.

"It was not intentional," my father said to me many years later when I brought it up. "Your mother and I were drunk at the time," he explained.

At the time, I knew they were drunk. That night, when they walked in the front door, I could smell the alcohol enter the space. I could see it in the way my mother could hardly stand. They were giddy and shushed each other. Then my father grabbed my mother's arm. "Ow, that hurts," she said. "Let go of me." Then she shook her arm loose.

The next thing I heard was a pop. My father formed a fist and, from the side, punched her in the face.

"I'll let go of you when I damn well feel like it," he said.

My mother winced. Her eyes clamped shut. And in slow motion, she lowered her head and brought her hands up. Then she cried into her open hands holding the pain.

"What did you do that for?" Her enunciation was muffled and sloppy. When she brought her hands back down, I saw blood.

"Mom! You're bleeding." I rushed over to her.

"Sit down," I said and directed her to the couch.

I went to the kitchen and grabbed a towel, drenched it in warm water, and ran back to her. I lifted her chin and gently placed the cloth over the blood. She turned her head away from me either out of pain or embarrassment.

"Let me clean you up," I said.

She reached for the towel.

"No, let me do it." I gently wiped the blood from her face. Her lip was swollen, but it was her nose that was bleeding. I got up and rushed to the bathroom and wadded toilet paper into a stopper and gently pushed it into each nostril just as she did for me when my nose bled. "Give me your hands?" I asked. I gently wiped the blood off and dried her hands with the other end of the towel.

My father staggered in with a little more skill and shouted, "She'll be fine."

He was drunk too. He darted for the bathroom and, without closing the door, pissed in the toilet. Then he crossed the hallway into his room and fell across the bed without taking off his clothes. I got up and closed the door behind him. Lately, I was doing that a lot. Closing the door after him. Separating him from the rest of us.

"Mom, sleep on the couch tonight," I said. I pulled the covers and pillow off my bed, ran back, and laid them next to her. I put the pillow on one end of the couch and helped her lie back. I removed her shoes and lifted her legs onto the cushions. Her legs were heavy. Each time I saw her like this my heart shattered. I wanted to help her, but I did not know how.

When I woke up the next morning, my mother and father were asleep, snuggled together in their bed. It was difficult for me to understand how they could hurt each other so violently and at the same time love each other so willingly.

8

KIRKBRIDE

I thought their drinking was the problem and all they had to do was stop. The drinking was a problem, but it covered up the real problem.

When my father drank, he was able to function. He never missed work. He never refused a second shift at work when offered. My mother, on the other hand, became progressively sad. In the middle of the day and without warning, she'd lose it. Her drive. Her appetite. Her understanding. She sat there aimlessly staring out the window. She was unreachable even when I stood in front of her asking what was wrong. She would not answer me.

As a child, I didn't know what to call it then, and as an adult, I still don't know what to call it now. But I witnessed the change that took over her mind. Her mood altered from complete happiness and fearlessness to absolute despair and unavoidable doom. When up, she was the perfect mom. When I returned from playing outside, she'd greet me at the front door with lemonade and a sandwich or a cookie. She was industrious and creative. With her sewing machine and scads of fabrics, she whipped together some of her most beautiful dresses. She made my brother's and my clothes. When I looked back at my childhood photographs, I was amazed at how skilled she was. The material that she used to make our pants was the same fabric on the cuffs and collars of our shirts. When she was up, she cooked and baked and kept a spotless house. She made joy for my brother and me with trips to the zoo, walks to the lake, and kite flying in the park. But when she was down, it was impossible to get her out of bed. And when she finally got up, she needed constant reassurance.

"Tell me how much you love me."

"Yes, you're the best, Mom." But she knew I was lying. She knew that I was worried. She knew that there was something wrong.

And then she started drinking. Maybe she was drinking the entire time, but it didn't affect her the way it was affecting her now. Sometimes the drinking smoothed out her mood swings. Sometimes the drinking made her sad and depressed. Sometimes she'd tell us that she did not want to live. Sometimes she threatened to kill herself.

Hearing those words frightened my father. Hearing those words frightened me. I didn't know what to make of it. What to do. However, he did.

He came to talk to me. He explained that Mom was sick and that he had to take her away to get help. When I asked where he was going, he said, "Kankakee." They got in the car, and she was gone for several weeks.

At the time, I didn't know what to make of it all. Kankakee sounded like a Native American name to me. Or maybe it was the name of her doctor. When she returned, she was sober and happy, and apologetic. She was more like the mom I remembered and more like the mom I wanted her to be. But it didn't last. The next day or the next week, and certainly by the next month, she was sad and drinking again.

Years later when I was in high school, I remembered what my father called it, Kankakee. I went to the library and looked it up. It is a city on the east bank of the Kankakee River in Illinois. In 1877, the Illinois legislature designated Kankakee as the site to build what at the time was called "a state hospital for the insane": a large complex with a soaring clock tower and two multistoried wings to the north and south. This asylum design was common throughout the mid- to late-nineteenth century. Thomas Kirkbride, a prominent Philadelphia psychiatrist, believed that appropriate architecture was integral to the treatment of mental illness. He believed that a healthy environment would heal an unstable mind. His goal was to remove patients with mental illness from overcrowded city jails where they were chained to the walls, and into buildings that provided ample sunlight and fresh air.

Kirkbride asylums were large, imposing, institutional buildings. The defining floor plan included a central building with long rambling wings in echelon that extended out from the center like wings on the body of a bat. Residence within the Kirkbride plan placed the most volatile and dangerous patients in sections farthest from the center. When my mother was institutionalized in the 1960s, I was not sure where she lived in the asylum.

When she returned home, my mother was better but still lonely. In 1962, instead of sending me to kindergarten like most five-year-olds, she kept me home with her. When I started first grade, it was a week late. During my time at home, I learned to take care of her, and she home-schooled me. I could read and my math skills were advanced. However, I also internalized her fears and anxieties. When I left for school in the morning, I worried that when I returned, I would not find her at home.

9

SECOND GRADE

In the front of the class, centered on the wall above the blackboard, was a large clock with a white dial and slender black hands. I watched that clock a lot. The hands ticked off the seconds and minutes and hours until it was time for me to go home. At 3:28 p.m., I stacked my reader and my speller in the upper left corner of my desk. I placed my writing pad and pencils on top of my books. I reached down on the left and retied the loose knot on my shoe. I pressed my heel deep into its inner sole, pulled the laces up tight, and quickly retied the ends. I did the same for the other shoe, but for this one, I doubled the knot. Then the bell rang. I stuffed my books and pencils into my satchel, leaped up from my desk, and dashed for the door.

"What's your rush, Mr. Lulich?" my second-grade teacher said while blocking the exit. Surely, she knew by now that I needed to get home. This was my daily routine.

"Mrs. Bell, my mother's expecting me to come home right away after school, please ma'am." I was attempting to squeeze between her and the way out. My hand flailed behind her back, searching for the doorknob. Finally, I grabbed it, turned it, unlatched the door, and slipped by her.

Parkside Elementary was a stately building of red brick and gray stone, a prime example of Palladian architecture, with strong symmetry, perspective lines, central arched windows, and false stone balconies above its main entrance. The three-story building with its flat roof sat in the center of the block, the girls' playground to the north and the boys' to the south, and the parameter fortified by a tall green wrought iron fence with straight bars spaced too narrow to slip between. That's how the government built schools in the early 1900s, impressive and imposing. The structure carried the weight of authority.

I lived at Sixty-Ninth and Cornell on Chicago's South Side. Parkside Elementary was on Sixty-Ninth and East End, the next street over. I barreled out the front door, ran north to Sixty-Ninth Street, made a left at the corner, ran west to Cornell Street, and then took another left. I rushed past my neighbors' houses, mostly single-story A-frame homes. Our urban block had sidewalks and front porches, small front yards, and a red fire hydrant that we kids illegally turned on to keep cool on hot summer days.

I would have made it home at breakneck speed if it wasn't for Mrs. Rainer. She lived near the corner, in the green frame house with the covered porch. It seemed as if she had a sixth sense about my whereabouts. She knew when I was out of the house, whether it was on school days or weekends, or when I just ran errands to the store for my mother. Maybe I am exaggerating, but it seemed that way. She wasn't mean or anything. But every time she saw me, she had to hug me and kiss me. Sometimes on my cheek, sometimes on my forehead, sometimes right on my mouth. It felt unnatural. My mother didn't even kiss me that way.

When I turned the corner onto Cornell Street rushing home from school that day, there she was. Impeccable timing and an obstacle that I had to overcome. Between me and reaching my mother was Mrs. Rainer. She was standing in the middle of the sidewalk with her arms outstretched to greet me. She looked more like a giant crab with big claws than a friendly neighbor. When I was close, she'd say my name repeatedly: "Jody, Jody, Jody," each succession more musical than the first. She'd smile, lean forward, and pucker her lips.

"Mrs. Rainer, I have got to get home, my mom is expecting me." Even I could hear my voice shake.

She'd say it again, "Jody, Jody, Jody," while sandwiching my face between her hands. She tilted my head up toward hers. As her face came in close to mine, the smell of her perfume went from floral to sickening. I shrank back in my body, closed my eyes, and wrinkled my nose. She planted one right on my mouth. Then she wrapped her claws around my body and hugged me while rocking me with her body in such an exaggerated fashion as if we were standing up in a canoe wavering back and forth before it tipped over.

I was short for my seven years and knew the only way out was down. With her bosoms resting on my head, I crouched down and wriggled until I squirmed right out of those claws, leaving her there with her arms supporting her chest. I darted off to the side and continued my dash home. Behind me, the musical echo of my name repeated over and over again. I didn't want to hurt her feelings. I was just not used to that type of affection. I turned around and said, "Sorry Mrs. Rainer, I have to get home. My mom needs me."

She responded, "Will I see you tomorrow?"

"I am sure you will," I said, too low for her to hear me. Then I waved and smiled, "Yes, I'll see you tomorrow, Mrs. Rainer. You will, you will, you will."

I turned back around, ran past several more houses and up the stairs of our front porch. I was careful not to grab on too tightly to that old wood banister.

My neck chain held the key to the front door. Before using it, I remembered that my mother said that I should knock or ring the doorbell first. She wanted to know that I made it home safely instead of just letting myself in and going to my room. Therefore, I knocked. And I waited. And I didn't hear anyone coming to let me in. I looked in the window. The house appeared unoccupied.

For the past three weeks, ever since school started, I hadn't had to use my key. My mother had been sober for almost a month. I knocked one more time. Then I let myself in.

"Mom, where are you?" I shouted.

Our first-floor duplex apartment was small, with a living room, dining room, bathroom, and kitchen on one side and, on the other side, two bedrooms in the back.

I walked in and shouted again, "Mom?"

The bathroom light was on. The door was partially open.

"Mom?" I said as I pushed the door in slowly. She was sitting on the toilet, passed out. Her panties were halfway down her legs. Her head and shoulders were slumped over the sink next to the toilet. Her face was resting on her arm.

"Mom," I said, this time nudging her leg back and forth several times.

"Huh," she said without lifting her head. The cigarette in her left hand between her fingers had extinguished itself. Ashes were on the floor.

"You could have burned down the house," I shouted.

"*Shush,* not so loud," she said, barely looking up at me. "Oh baby, I would never do that. I would never do anything to hurt you." Her words were slurred and inaudible at the end. I could smell the liquor on her breath. I was worried because my father would be home soon.

"Mom, you're drunk," I hollered.

"I'm not; I just had one glass."

I had no time to argue. "Dad's going to be home soon, and I need to get you in bed. Let's go. Lean against me?"

She did not move. I put one arm over my left shoulder and her other arm over my right shoulder. "Put your hands together around my neck and pull yourself up."

Nothing. I lightly slapped the side of her face to rouse her.

"What?" she said and grabbed my hand to stop.

"Put your hands around my neck and pull yourself up. I have got to get you to bed."

"Oh baby, okay."

When she pulled herself up, I pulled her panties up to her waist. I left her pants on the bathroom floor.

"Lean against me. I need to get you to bed. Dad will be home soon." It wasn't pretty, but we made it across the hall and onto her side of the bed. I wish that I had removed the covers first. I went to the other side and rolled up the covers close to her. Then I rolled her to the other side onto the sheets. She flopped over perfectly. Her head landed on the pillow. I removed her shoes and placed them under the bed as if she had taken them off herself. "Mom, put your arms above your head." Again, no response. "Mom I need you to help me; put your arms above your head." She didn't budge, but she didn't resist. I pulled her blouse up over her head and off. I went to the dresser and removed a nightgown. I rolled up the garment and easily slipped it over her head. Then I put her left arm through the sleeve. I rolled her slightly on her back, freeing her right arm. Then I put her right arm through the other sleeve. I tried to pull the nightgown down as far as possible, but when I reached her hips, she was dead weight. I finally pulled the covers over her. "It's going to be all right, Mom," I said. I went to the kitchen and grabbed a small linen cloth. I ran water over one corner until it was damp. I opened the toothpaste and smeared some on the cloth.

"Mom, stick your tongue out." I reached in and wiped her tongue. She jerked back, coughed, and I removed my hand before she clamped her teeth over my fingers.

"What are you doing?" she scolded.

You are up now, I thought.

"You're drunk. You smell drunk. Dad's going to be home soon. I am trying to clean you up."

"Just leave me alone," she said as her arm went up and pushed me away.

This time I only lifted her lips and wiped the outside of her gums and teeth.

I opened the closet and threw the cloth down the laundry chute. I took her brush from the top of the dresser and brushed her hair.

"Mom," I whispered. "It's going to be okay. But you have got to stop drinking. Promise me you'll stop."

"Stop what, baby?"

"Stop drinking."

"I told you that I only had one glass."

"Mom, just promise me that you'll stop. Promise!"

"Okay, Hon, I will stop." And she fell back asleep. I stood there a while and looked at her. I looked at her and looked at her as if looking at her would change her. Would change her into what I wanted her to be, into what I wanted us to be. And then, I stopped looking.

I rushed to the bathroom and cleaned up the mess. I picked her cigarette butt off the floor and threw it in the toilet. I scrubbed the sink and toilet with cleanser. And then I scrubbed the floor. When I was done, it was beginning to smell more like bleach than booze.

Then I went to the kitchen. "Mom, what were you going to cook for dinner?" I shouldn't have bothered asking. She was passed out. I opened the refrigerator. On the door—butter, mayonnaise, mustard, and ketchup. On the first shelf—milk, water, and orange juice. On the shelf below—pickles, eggs, bread. The drawer on the left—oranges, apples, carrots, celery; I hated celery. In the right drawer—chicken. I knew how to cook chicken. I took it out and set it on the sink. I pushed in the knob in the center of the stove and turned on the gas. I opened the box of matches on the top of the stove, opened the oven door. Struck the match. It took several strikes, and then the match lit. I placed it near the small round opening on the floor of the oven. *Vooosh!* the match ignited the burner and the excess gas in the oven. A large flame flew out and vanished just as quickly but not before singing my eyelashes. I must remember not to do that again.

I turned the flame down and closed the oven door. I washed the chicken and patted it dry. I pulled a pan out and lined it with aluminum foil. I placed the pieces of chicken in the pan, sprinkled salt and pepper over the top, and put it in the oven. I grabbed four potatoes, one for each of us, washed them, and pierced their skin several times with a fork. I put them in the oven next to the chicken. Then I finished cleaning. On the counter, I spotted the empty bottle and the glass from which she had been drinking. I rinsed out the glass, dried it, and put it away on the top shelf of the cabinet. I took the bottle outside to the large garbage drum in the alley. I dropped it in, reached down as far as I could, and covered the bottle with trash. As I came in the back door, the front door opened, and my father walked in. He saw the dining room table. It was set for only three, and he asked, "Where is your brother?"

"I don't know. I haven't seen Gary all day," I said.

"Dad, Mom isn't feeling well. She set the table just for us and Gary and put dinner in the oven and asked me to take it out in an hour. I think she has a headache or something. She looked tired and went to bed."

He sat down on the couch, rubbed his forehead with his hand, using his fingers to massage away the tension. Then he picked up the mail. He was quiet, dinner was quiet, and the evening was quiet.

When my brother returned much later, and I went to bed, I heard my mother and father arguing. It was calm, compared with their usual fights. They were trying to argue without letting us hear. But I was familiar with the low tones and curt phrases of my father's admonishing voice and the shrill tones of my mother's denials. You didn't have to make out the words to know that they were at it again.

I tried to fall asleep, but all I could do was feel sorry for my mother. She was too drunk to understand how angry my father was. She was too drunk to understand that he needed to be heard—even as he slowed the pace and took his time—even when his words were kind and loving. And that early phase of my father being somewhat sympathetic, then impatient, was fast leading to more drastic responses.

10

SECOND SHIFT

My father worked swing shifts at General Mills. When he worked the first shift, we all got up early in the morning. As my father got ready for work, my brother and I got ready for school. When my father sat down to eat breakfast, we ate breakfast with him. He left for work before we left for school, but we returned home two hours before he returned from work. When my father worked the first shift, we ate dinner as a family, all four of us around the same table.

When my father worked the second shift, we didn't actually see him for that week. When we left for school, he was asleep. We were quiet in the morning so as not to disturb him. He left for work before we came home. He returned at midnight after my brother and I were already in bed.

Third shift was the midnight shift. My father left for work after my brother and I went to bed. He returned in the morning when we were leaving for school.

Working a different shift every week was not easy on him and it was not easy on us. But of all the shifts, second shift was the most treacherous.

*

I woke up in the middle of the night to the sound of smashing glass. Then my father shouted, "This is the last time."

Next, I heard my mother apologizing repeatedly, "I'm sorry. I'm sorry." Her words were slurred. I knew why. She was drunk. Again.

My brother and I slept in the same room. He was awake too. He placed his finger to his lips and signaled for me to be quiet. When he saw me push back the covers, he motioned me to stop. I ignored him. I got out of bed and walked through the kitchen. I stopped at the doorjamb before entering their space.

My father sat at the dining room table. Green peas, mashed potatoes, and pieces of chicken were strewn over one side of the floor. Fragments of a broken dinner plate littered the space. A shattered glass of milk covered the dispersed meal like gravy. Food splattered against the wall oozed down to the floor. It looked as if my father had hurled his entire dinner against the wall in one monumental stroke.

My mother knelt on the floor; she was bent over the wreckage. With her apron tied around her waist, she folded up its bottom edge to form a pocket that she filled with broken glass and bits of food.

My father, fuming, sat erect. The muscles on his lower jaw were throbbing. He kept his mouth closed and breathed heavily through his nose. Then, without warning, he abruptly stood up. And when he did, his chair toppled to the floor behind him.

I stepped back into the shadow of the kitchen.

My father repeated himself, "This is the last time." He stepped behind my mother, reached down, and grabbed her wrist. He swung her arm out and then twisted it up behind her back. She winced and shifted her feet beneath her body, struggling to rise and release the tension on her arm. And when she did, food and broken glass fell from her apron and hit the floor a second time.

My father stepped toward her and pinned her against the wall. With his other hand, he grabbed the back of her collar and pulled her upper body close to him. "This is the last time," he repeated at a slow steady pace through clenched teeth.

Again, she tried to stay standing. She rose up on her toes to ease the pain shooting through her arm. In doing so, she looked up and saw me standing under the archway at the entrance to the dining room. My father followed her line of sight and caught me watching as the events unfolded.

"Go back to your room and close the door," he screamed.

I did not budge. I hoped that my presence would make my father stop hurting her. But he didn't let go of her. He wrenched her arm farther up her back. My mother sobbed, helpless. Her body trembled as tears fell across her cheeks.

"Call the police," she said in a rush.

I turned around and grabbed the receiver from the telephone on the kitchen wall. I pressed it against my ear and placed my hand over the dial.

My father watched my every move. He lessened his grip, but never let go.

In a clear and deliberate voice, he shouted, "Put the phone down."

I closed my eyes for reasons that I cannot explain. But when I opened them, nothing had changed. The telephone was still in my hand. My mother was still struggling to stay upright. My father, angrier than ever, still pinned her against the wall, with his body twisting her arm behind her back.

My father grabbed her collar again, this time winding it around his hand. *He's choking her,* I thought.

"Put down the phone," he said again, this time each word striking me like punches to my face.

I did not know what to do. I knew my mother was drunk. I knew my father had worked all evening and was tired. I knew he was in control, or maybe out of control. Every time he yanked her arm, she screamed. And every time she screamed, I shuddered.

Then she looked deep into my eyes. I looked back and gave her my full attention. She stopped sobbing. She was in extreme pain, but her face relaxed. It became soft and she relented. Then she nodded and with her gaze, she set me free. If a look could be articulated, she was saying I should not call the police.

I opened my hand. The receiver fell to the floor.

My father yanked her away from the wall and dragged her backward to the front door. The rustling sound of her feet rubbing against the carpet as she struggled to stay upright left me breathless. Although she released me, I still feared for her.

My father shoved her around in the opposite direction and rammed her body against the front door. The windows rattled. Then he pulled her back into him, turned the knob, and opened the door. A blast of cold air blew in. With the door wide open, he shoved her out into the bitter freezing night and slammed the door behind her. I heard the latch click as he locked the door.

11

FALLING

When I sleep, I dream. And when I dream, I dream of flying. I am a great blue heron. My ascent is slow. My stroke is expansive. I begin as if I were swimming through air. I reach forward, sweep my arms out and back. I lift and my feet leave the floor. I beat my feet in unison like the large tail fluke of a dolphin and rise.

In my dream, the ceiling, and the attic, and the roof of my house are a translucent gel. I look up and see the moon shining down. With my hands extending up over my head, I beat my foot, rise, and pierce the ceiling.

Up here, it is quiet. I am safe.

I look down into the house. My father enters through the front door. Dirty dishes are piled in the kitchen sink, and spoiled food rots in the refrigerator. My mother leans in to greet him. Her odd but familiar cloying stench fills his nostrils. He steps back because he knows she is drunk. Each volatile exhale provokes his disapproval. When she gets within arm's length, his right hand lands hard against the left side of her face. A loud crack. She sucks her lower lip in and tastes the blood trickling inside her mouth. Before she utters an apology, *Crack!* My father, using the same hand, reverses direction and strikes her again. The unexpected blow throws her off balance. She steadies herself, a feat no ordinary drunkard could have accomplished without practice. But the pain lingers. The closing of her eyes follows the inward collapse of her face. She raises her hand to hold her head. This unexpected gesture blocks a third strike from his other hand and leaves her with enough sensibility and time to run to the bathroom and lock the door. The living room grows dark.

Up here, I am safe, but I am disgusted at both of them.

I look down again. A soft yellow glow illuminates the kitchen. We sit around a small table in the middle of the room. We are enjoying dinner. My mother and father sit facing each other. I sit on the opposite side of the table from my brother. He is only an arm's length away but uses his foot to make contact. He lifts his leg and kicks the front of mine. I have learned to ignore his provocations. I have learned to ignore him entirely. So he kicks harder. I avoid eye contact or any indication of pain and keep eating. My resolve agitates him. He slouches down in his chair, positions his foot closer. His next kick, harder than any previous, delivers a sloppy blow. He misses me and hits the dog, who squeals like a mouse and runs from under the table. I feel sorry for our dog and wish that I had taken the blow. My father, using both fists, pounds the table. He demands to know "who started it?" Before either can deliver an explanation, he slaps us both. My eyes close because I do not want to see anymore.

When I do open them, I peer down into my parents' bedroom. The room is dark except for a reflection of the moon peering through sheer curtains. The moon's glow is white, metallic in its hue. The entire room takes on the same steely harshness. My parents lie awake in bed. The light seeping into the room casts faint shadows over their faces. My mother and father lie facing away from each other. Only an arm's length apart, the chasm between them is infinite. She teeters off the edge of the bed closest to the door. She knows that this is the fastest escape route. He feels betrayed because money is spent on alcohol while dinner goes unprepared and food in the refrigerator spoils. Under these circumstances, neither will sleep tonight.

The front porch light comes on and I watch as the front door opens. I see them leave. The door closes. My father enters on the driver's side of our iconic 1957 four-door beige Chevy. My mother takes her time but eventually enters on the passenger side. In this beefy car with winged fenders above the rear wheels and a cormorant hood ornament, they sit on the same seat an arm's length away, but miles apart. He starts the engine, steers away from the curb, and drives into the night. From high in the sky like a bird I swoop down and follow the car. I cannot hear their conversation, but their frantic breathing and strained facial expressions define their disgust with each other. When the car reaches the corner, it turns right and travels south. They drive through Jackson Park toward Lake Michigan. Theirs is the only car on the road. The headlights pierce the night, projecting cones of yellow light on the road ahead. Just as the car turns right, to enter the freeway, a larger car speeding in the cross street slams into the side of their car. With uncompromising force, the 1957 Chevy is hit hard. Instead of collapsing around the point of impact, the car heaves up and tumbles over and off the road. It tumbles through the safety barricade. It tumbles into the lake and sinks. Air from the cabin gurgles to the surface, releasing bursts of hostility. Then there is silence. Nothing else rises. Not hope. Not remorse. Not forgiveness.

Nothing rises until the police come. They shine their lights on the lake's reflecting surface. Divers put oxygen tanks on their backs, goggles over their eyes, regulators in their mouths, and dive like ducks below the surface. First, they drag my mother out and place her on the shore. Her breathing has ceased. Her mouth is tightly closed. Minutes later, my father is heaved up. His condition is identical. They are positioned on the shore, parallel to each other and only an arm's length apart. The officer shines a flashlight on their faces. Both are ashen.

In the days that follow, they are buried as they were placed on the shore, next to each other, in individual graves an arm's length apart. If only someone had repositioned their hands and carefully uncoiled my father's fingers until his fists relaxed into an open palm. If someone had pulled down my mother's arms from shielding her face and placed them at her sides, my parents would have appeared happy as if they were part of a family, as if they cared for each other.

The night's sky could hold no more sorrow. As the moon set and the sun rose, the horizon transformed into infinite, vertical gradients of color from black to blue to burnt orange.

I am exhausted and begin falling. And when I look down, I see my brother below me anxiously shaking his fists at me. I struggle to stay up. My arms flap frantically as I grab for the air above me. I twist left and then right to gain height. But I keep sinking. First through the roof. Then through the attic. Then my foot moves in and out of my bedroom ceiling. My brother climbs on the bed and jumps in the air to catch me. His hand swipes the side of my foot but doesn't take hold. He lands without me. He bends his knees, crouches down, and with one enormous heave, leaps into the air. He rises and hooks both hands tightly around my ankles. I jerk my legs, but he holds on. With the weight of his body, he whips me out of the air and onto my bed. I land on my back. Air gushes out of my lungs. He pounces on top and straddles his legs along the sides of my hips. He shoves the meat of his palms over my shoulders and pins me down. I sink deep into the mattress. "Why did you kill them?" he shouts.

"It is a dream," I tell him.

I struggle to get him off me. He is big and I am small. He is strong and I am weak. But he is right.

He jerks me up and thrusts me back down. I help him. I deserve whatever he delivers. Then with all his might, he shoves me down hard. The bed cracks open and we fall. We fall through the floor. We fall past my mother and father arguing, past the 1957 Chevy at the bottom of the lake. We fall past the point where light cannot penetrate. While falling, he realizes that all we have left is each other. He reaches for me, this time without malice and without hatred. He holds me. He holds me as if he understands me. I wrap my arms around his waist and press deep into him. I hold him as tightly as I can until there's nothing between us. Not air. Not water. Not light. Not time. Not animosity and not regret. And I answer him, "They were hurting each other. I wanted it to stop."

12

CHRISTMAS EVE, 1966

As darkness blanketed our street, one by one the neighbors' houses light up in brilliant colors of red and green and white and blue. In their front windows, Christmas trees twinkled with blinking lights and sparkling tinsel. Decorative garlands covered handrails leading to front porches. Pine wreaths with red bows and red berries hung from doors. Strings of multicolored lights framed windows. Plastic Santas with red cheeks and big bellies glowed on front porches. One house had a wood cutout of life size reindeers and a sleigh filled with toys. All the way down the street every house was lit up with Christmas decorations, except ours.

Many things were different that Christmas. My father was rarely home. And when he was, he avoided my mother. He spent his time in the basement organizing his tools, putting spare screws in jars and loose nails in boxes. He attached pegboard to the wall and hung up his screwdrivers, his wire cutters and hammers, and his hacksaws and coping saws. He fixed things that were broken. He repaired the agitator in our old Kenmore washing machine. He fixed the squeaky belt that rotated the drum of the clothes dryer. He rewired motors that no longer revved. He did not deal with what he could not fix.

That same holiday week, my mother spent most of her time in bed. She stopped washing our clothes and changing our bed covers. She cooked dinner but left it on the stove for us to dish up and feed ourselves. For a while, she still enjoyed sewing. She was making a jacket for herself, but after a few days, her sewing machine sat silent and collected dust. Pieces of fabric piled up around its legs. A swatch of burgundy corduroy and the tape side of a black zipper were perpetually locked under the sewing machine's presser foot, the sewing needle driven through both fabrics as if the electricity had gone off in mid-stitch.

My brother spent his time with his friends. His trips home in the evenings were to eat dinner and sleep in his bed, and sometimes he didn't come home for that.

I tried to help my mother. After dinner, I packed up the leftover food and put it in the refrigerator. I cleaned the dishes. After drying the dishes, I put them away in the cabinet. I washed clothes and made sure that there were clean towels in the bathroom. When it snowed, I picked up the broom and swept off the porch and the front stairs.

In the evening, I read to her. I was in the middle of *The Call of the Wild,* by Jack London. The main character, Buck, a powerful sled dog, is stolen from his family in California, forcibly transported to the Canadian wilderness, and trained for hard labor. When Buck is about to be beaten, John Thornton prevents the trainer from hurting Buck and sets him free. From then on Buck works only for John and never leaves his side.

I went into my mother's room, sat on the floor at the foot of her bed, and read aloud. When I read the section where John Thornton says, "I love you, Buck," I looked up at my mother. She lifted her head and her eyes opened. She looked back at me. I paused. I wanted her to invite me to sit on the bed next to her. I wanted her to say that she loved me as John Thornton said he loved Buck. Instead, a long silence separated us. Then she lay back down and closed her eyes. I leaned against the side of her bed and continued reading, this time softer and slower.

After my mother fell asleep, I walked back to the living room and looked out the window. Snow was falling. I put on my coat. When I opened the door, my brother was on the outside reaching for the doorknob. I wanted to ask where he had been but did not. Besides, my preteen twelve-year-old brother would never tell his little nine-year-old brother where he had been all evening. On my way out, I asked him to please not lock the door.

"I'm just going on the porch," I told him. "I just want to sit outside for a while."

"In the cold?" he questioned me.

"Yeah," I said. "You want to join me?"

"Nope," my brother said.

I stepped aside to let him pass. On my way out, I turned back around and reminded him, "Please don't lock the door. It's cold and I do not have my keys."

I sat down on the top step of our porch. Thick snow collected on my eyelashes and eyebrows. I looked down the street. I could see inside our neighbors' houses. Children were dancing. In another house, they were playing tag. Living rooms were full of excitement and anticipation. Everyone around us seemed happy.

I thought about a time when we were happy. In the winter, we would walk to the outdoor ice-skating rink at the Midway. My brother and I were bundled up in matching blue snowsuits. Our parents tied the laces of their ice skates together and draped them over their shoulders or around their necks. Mom and Dad walked ahead of us, holding each other's hand. Gary and I were behind in the sled, hitchhiking a ride to the rink. Our father held the bridle tightly as he pulled us over snowbanks. When we reached the rink, Mom and Dad put on their skates. Our mother raced to the rink while my brother and I sat on a snowbank and watched. Mom was skillful. She skated with the grace and speed of a cheetah. First forward and then backward, weaving between the other skaters. Spotting us, she would wink, take in a full breath of air and dart away, hurling flakes of surface ice into the air. Then it was Dad's turn. What he lacked in grace, he made up for in speed. He nodded at us, letting us know that he was going after her and would be back shortly. He raced to the rink as steam rose beneath his heavy scarf. Darting through the crowd, he spotted her. It was no longer an exhibition of skill, but speed. My father was faster. He quickly caught up and swallowed her into his arms. Unable to shift their momentum and adjust their balance, they both came crashing to the ice, sliding completely across the rink until stopped by the snowbank at our feet. We all laughed. After taking off his skates, my father lifted me from the snow and carried me on his back. My arms were wrapped tightly around his neck. My brother pulled the sled as we all walked home, bumping into one another with the sides of our bodies and giggling.

I lowered my head into my cupped hands and closed my eyes. It was Christmas Eve and we didn't have a Christmas tree. There would be no gifts. My parents were not speaking to each other. Tomorrow, dinner would be nothing special. I would likely eat alone in the bedroom or in front of the TV.

I was cold. I lifted the hood on the back of my coat and pulled it over my head. "It's okay," I said to myself.

I opened my eyes and looked down the street one more time. It was beautiful, a kaleidoscope of colors. I stood up, turned around, twisted the doorknob, and opened the door. I smiled. My brother remembered to leave it unlocked.

I stepped in and took off my coat. I rubbed my hands together to warm my fingers and then stuffed them into the pockets of my pants. When I looked up, my brother was standing in the middle of the living room on a sturdy chair from the kitchen. With Scotch tape in one hand and a silver-colored star in the other, he was attaching our Christmas tree ornaments to the living room ceiling. There were shiny bells and metallic balls and bows of every color. There were clowns and spinning tops. He hung the angels playing trumpets and the snowmen with carrot noses. There were Santas and sleigh bells. There were reindeer, horses, cats, and dogs. There were silver art deco pine cones and real pine cones with glitter that dangled from red string. He hung the snowflakes woven from straw and the snowflakes knitted from yarn. There was tinsel in his hair and tinsel on the floor. He filled every space on the ceiling with ornaments. Then he strung the Christmas tree lights over the archways and windows.

I wanted to thank him. I wanted to stand in front of him, lean forward, and rest my forehead on his chest. I wanted to wrap my arms around him. But after plugging in the colored lights, he picked up the chair and set it back at the kitchen table. And when I turned around, he was already in the bedroom that we shared in the back of the house. I started to follow him, but I kept turning around and looking at the ceiling. I could not take my eyes off all the ornaments. I lay down on my back in the middle of the floor. I kept looking up, thinking how wonderful. Some of the ornaments I had made in school. Some had been in our family for as long as I could remember. I remembered hanging them on last year's Christmas tree.

Then the doorbell rang. When I opened the door, standing in front of me was Mrs. Rainer. She wore a heavy coat with a fur collar and a big smile. "Merry Christmas," she said and handed me two boxes. "One is for you and one is for your brother," she said. I reached over and hugged her. "I have to go and deliver more presents," she said. "Don't open them until tomorrow."

"I promise," I said and nodded at the same time. As she walked down the stairs, I called out, "Merry Christmas, Mrs. Rainer."

I would have lain back down in the middle of the floor, but instead, I went to the front window. I opened the curtains as wide as I could. I tied them back to keep them open. I wanted all of our neighbors to see the ornaments hanging from the ceiling and the lights over the windows. I wanted them to know that my brother made our Christmas without a tree and toys, without hot apple cider, and without turkey and cranberry sauce.

When I think back on that Christmas Eve, it is difficult for me to not cry. Mrs. Rainer's presents—a jigsaw puzzle and a paint-by-number kit—were the only gifts we received. The best gift, however, was my brother's thoughtfulness. He expressed a tenderness that I had never experienced before and at a time when it was sorely needed. He left an enormous impression on me that night, a thumbprint on my heart where only his finger fits and unlocks this simple and wondrous memory.

13

NEW YEAR'S EVE, 1966

That was the night my father armed himself with a weapon I suspect that he will regret using the rest of his life. After smashing his wedding ring with that sledgehammer, he threw the ring at my mother and shouted at her to get out of his life.

That was the night my mother got out of bed, went to the kitchen, removed a container from under the sink, filled a glass, and drank it. When she got back in bed and lifted the covers, my father's mutilated wedding ring fell to the floor. That was the last sound I heard all night.

When my father returned the next morning, my mother was unmistakably ill. She refused to tell my father what she had done. He asked if I knew anything and I said no. My father searched the house, opening drawers and closets. When he found an opened bottle of antifreeze under the kitchen sink, he and my brother carried her to the car and rushed her to the hospital. They left me at home alone. Lying in bed, I wondered if I would ever see my mother again.

Sometime between midnight and daybreak, I heard a car door shut and I opened my eyes. It was dark inside the house and dark outside. Then I heard a second car door shut. I forced my body out of bed. Whatever the outcome, I had to begin to make sense of it. I needed to know, but also feared what I might be told.

I pushed the covers back from over my head and my legs. I sat up on the edge of the bed. I extended my feet down and placed them on the floor. I braced my legs beneath me and stood up.

I heard house keys press into the lock of the front door. The deadbolt released.

I ran out of the bedroom toward the front of the house. I walked through the dining room. Then I stopped. I could go no farther. I stood motionless in the space between the dining room and the living room, the wide gap that separated my wildest thoughts from unavoidable reality. I froze. I stared at the front door, now only ten feet in front of me.

Any other time, the door would have swung open as soon as the key released the lock. The door did not swing open. I waited. Thirty seconds. Then a minute. Maybe longer. Then the door opened slowly. Dark shadows poured over the living room floor and billowed toward me.

From that unexpected delay it took for the door to open, I knew. When my father stepped out of the darkness and into the dimly lit living room, from his slow tentative walk, and the shallow look on his face, I knew. From the awkward tilt of his head and the narrowing of his eyes as if he were searching for the words and how to position them just right before telling me, I knew. When he didn't kneel and stretch open his arms to catch me as I started to come toward him, I knew. So I hesitated. I drew inward and kept my distance. When my uncle Marty, my father's brother, whom I had not seen for months, entered from the same darkness, immediately after my father, I knew. My brother, who entered the house next, who would chide me regardless of the circumstance, now was quiet and gentle, I knew. I knew, because after he entered, the door closed behind him, evaporating any hope that my mother would step out from the darkness and into the light of the living room to greet me. I knew.

My father took in a slow deep breath, his body stiffened, and my body stiffened as I braced myself. However, his mouth remained shut. He slowly exhaled without parting his lips. As his cheeks filled with air, I imagined all the things that he wanted to tell me. *Don't drag this out. . . ,* I wanted to scream. *Tell me. Just tell me.* He hesitated. And then all the air trapped in his inflated cheeks escaped through his nose with an audible hiss as his face flattened and his shoulders lowered.

My eyes teared up. It made no sense to delay what I already knew. If he could only read my face, he would understand that I needed to hear it. I needed to hear something. Anything.

We looked at each other. He blinked several times. Then my father took in another long, full resonating breath through his nose that completely filled his chest. As he exhaled, his mouth opened, and his words came out like chunks of ice that fell to the floor and shattered into a million pieces. I was not prepared to hear what he just said even though I already knew.

I imagined that my father would take me through the evening as it happened. He would tell me that they arrived at the hospital at breakneck speed. My father would tell me that the doctors quickly admitted her. That the doctors were smart and knew exactly what to do. He would tell me that they cured her vomiting. That my mother wondered where I was. That she loved me. That she would get better. That she was sorry for putting us through this again. That she made a horrible mistake. I wanted to hear that my mother would recover. And while telling me these things, I needed my father to kneel down and hold me, and whisper in my ear that he understood how difficult this was for me. That I would not be alone. I needed him to say that regardless of what happens, he would never leave me.

That is not what happened. My father did not hold me. Instead, he put distance between us. He averted his gaze. He said that what he had to tell me was important, but he could not tell me any more until I promised.

Promise? Promise what, I thought. Why is he putting me through this? I was confused. What did it matter if I promised or not? Then he repeated himself, I need you to promise. I slowly nodded. Then he said it fast, "I need you to promise not to cry."

It was as if a wall of glass came up from the floor, slicing the air between us, sealing me from sound, and love, and hope. All night I had been preparing myself for the worst, but I did not expect this.

Trembling, I said, "I promise."

Even now as an adult, I do not understand why I promised. I knew what he had to tell me, and I promised anyway, a promise that would protect him and leave me vulnerable and questioning if my feelings mattered at all. A promise that would damage my relationship with my father for the rest of our lives. He had his brother, my uncle Marty, and my brother for support, and I had no one. I looked up at him for an instant. His mouth opened. I saw his lips move. I heard him whisper my name.

"Jody."

At that instant, I drew back my love. I watched his mouth open and his lips move, but I stopped hearing. I looked down at the floor. I focused on my mother. When I looked back up at him, his last three words were unmistakable.

His lips gently came together and then briefly parted with a short puff of air before closing, forming the word MOM.

Then his jaw and bottom lip slightly lowered as minuscule droplets of moisture hurled out before he loosely closed his mouth, forming the word IS.

Finally, with his lips slightly parted, I saw his tongue rise behind the tips of his upper teeth and then lower to the bottom of his mouth before slowly returning upward, stretching his final word, DEAD, from what was normally a single short syllable into what I imagined was a long resonating echo.

My father's upper body collapsed beneath his shirt, revealing the tremendous effort these final words took from him, and from me. My eyes closed. I swallowed to clear saliva collecting in the back of my throat.

At nine, I was the youngest. At nine, my eyes were level with the buckle of my father's belt. That was my focus, an inanimate object of no concern. *I need to keep standing,* I told myself.

I kept perfectly still, but my eyes could not hide how I felt. They darted from side to side searching for support from anyone in the room. Then they remained steady and opened as wide as possible. They welled up with tears, so I knew not to shut them. If I shut them, tears would fall down my cheeks.

I looked up at my father, hoping that he would rescind his request, hoping that he would reach down, pick me up, and hold me. I hoped that he would realize that I needed his support as much as he needed mine. His position never changed.

On the inside, I was breaking into pieces. I teetered on the verge of collapse.

On the outside, I remained standing. I stood for him. I stood because my mother would have wanted me to. I tightened my fists and anchored my feet. I willed my body to stand straight. And when I finally closed my eyes, because I had to close my eyes to hold it together, not one tear fell.

14

THE ACCIDENT

The morning of my mother's funeral, the sun struggled to break through the clouds. A bluish-gray hue covered everything from the trees to the sidewalks, from the snow-covered rooftops to the snow-covered lawns, from the reflections off windows of every parked car and every still house. This worrisome shade of gray hung there and consumed everything I saw.

I opened my closet, looked at my clothes, and thought, *What color is anger?* Red flashed in my mind.

If a car had hit my mother, I would have been angry at the driver. If she had had cancer, I would have been angry at God. But my mother did this to herself, and I was angry at her. I looked back in my closet. Not a red shirt in the bunch.

Should I wear a blue shirt? What shade of blue is loss? What color is regret?

I slid an undershirt over my head and pulled it down over my belly and back. Over it, I fastened a gray, long-sleeve shirt. I buttoned it all the way up to my chin. Then I yanked a pair of black pants off a hanger. I stepped into them, pulled them up, and fastened them around my waist. I was shaking. I was cold. I put my arms into an over-sized brown cardigan sweater. The sleeves dangled past my wrists. I slid my sleeves up. I saw my fingernails that I had bitten down to the nub.

Dressed, I picked up my winter coat and dragged myself to the living room. I fell into the couch, dropped my coat to my side, and slumped over the armrest. I turned my head up and looked into what was now an empty house.

Later, when my father walked into the living room, I was still slumped over on my side. He asked if I wanted to eat something. I said that I was not hungry. He went to the refrigerator, walked back, and dropped a red apple in my lap. I did not look up. I did not say thank you. I looked past him, squinting and staring into the house. He walked away without saying another word.

When my brother got out of bed, I heard him rearranging the hangers in the closet and picking up the ones that I had knocked to the floor. We shared the same closet. His clothes were on one side and mine were on the other. He would know what to wear. He walked out of the bedroom in dark pants and a white shirt. Neither of us owned a suitcoat or a necktie. Neither of us had a reason to. Neither of us had been to a funeral before.

When my father and brother were ready to leave, they waved at me to follow. I sat there, resisting.

"Hey, it is time to go," my father said as he made his way out the front door.

I stood up from the couch. The red apple fell from my lap and tumbled across the floor. I put my arms into my brown parka, shoving the back of it up and over my shoulders. I picked up the apple and stuffed it in my coat pocket. Before closing the door, I turned around and looked in. My mother's sewing machine was silent and dusty. The red jacket she had started was still under the presser foot, the fabric falling to the floor.

Parked out front was our blue station wagon, already three years old and dirty from hauling around building materials to fix our house. We climbed in. My father sat up front behind the steering wheel. My brother sat in the passenger seat behind him. I sat across from my brother, as far to the right as possible, and directly behind where my mother would have sat if she were with us.

As the car pulled away from the curb, I regretted getting up and getting dressed. I didn't want to go. I kept turning around and look-ing at our house. As the car moved forward, the facade of our porch with its brown steps and wood railing became smaller and smaller until it disappeared among the other porches on our block. Then I turned around and faced the road. I leaned against the inside of the passenger door, lowered my head, and closed my eyes.

Our drive was silent. The scrunching sound of snow packing beneath the tires of our car was all I heard for most of the drive.

Silence was how my father dealt with disappointment. Silence was how I learned to deal with it too. However, the uncertainty as to what would happen to me and my brother frightened me. I worried about who would take care of us now that our mother was gone. When my mother went to Kankakee to recuperate, we slept at our grandmother's house. The day after our mother's death, we spent several nights at Aunt Cleo's with our cousins. I needed to know what happens to children when their mother dies. *Would our father keep us?*

We came to the end of our block and turned left. When we reached the next corner, the streetlight turned red. We stopped. We waited, but no cars crossed. When the light turned green, we sped up and continued on our way. Ahead, a group of kids played kickball in the street. They were playing to win. Steam jetted out from their noses. When our car came close, they continued their game. We slowed down. Finally, a taller boy picked up the ball, suspending the action. The other boys moved to either side of the street and opened a path for us. We drove through. As we moved between them, the smallest boy waved to me. He must have recognized the sorrow on my face. I waved but could not smile. After we passed, the ball flew into the air. The boys quickly repositioned themselves on the pavement and restarted the game. I admired their carefree risk-taking by playing in the street. I envied their ability to have fun and not worry about life's unexpected turns.

Several blocks later, we approached a tree-lined street. The wind picked up. The trees were bare. Their branches swayed and played with the daylight over the road ahead. Then, from out of nowhere, a large dog darted out of an alley and sprinted toward our car. He was lean and muscled. He had a dense coat of dark-brown fur, erect ears, a narrow snout, and large dark-brown eyes. He looked well cared for and street smart, and as if he could outrun any car. As we got closer, the dog sped up. I worried and braced my hands against the back of the seat in front of me. I knew that once my father saw him, he would slam on the brakes. I was used to my father slamming on the brakes. The kids on my block always played in the street. My dad was a careful driver. However, this time was different. My father's mind was elsewhere, maybe focused on the funeral, maybe thinking how he will care for Gary and me. Maybe on regret. The moment my father caught sight of that sprinting dog, it was too late. The dog also misjudged our approach. Our car hit the dog and the dog disappeared under the front bumper. All of him, his thick brown coat, his erect ears, his large dark-brown eyes. Our car jerked up and down before returning to smooth pavement. I wasn't sure if we drove over a rut in the road or our wheels ran over the well-muscled dog. I turned around and looked out the back window. The dog lay motionless in the middle of the street, his head yanked back in an unnatural position.

At first, my father slowed down. For a millisecond, he looked startled. I looked at my father from behind. I could see his face in the rearview mirror. He looked down and glanced at his wristwatch. His eyes returned to the road and our car continued onward.

If my father had spotted me in the rearview mirror, he would have seen the worry on my face. He would have seen my mouth open as I gasped in disbelief. A car barreling down the road on the other side of the street didn't stop either. It was as if this dog's life meant nothing. I sank lower in my seat, closed my eyes, and put my hands over my face.

When our car pulled up outside the funeral home, I slowly lifted my head and straightened my back. I watched as families made their way in the front door. Women wore long dark-wool coats with animal-fur collars. Men wore dark suitcoats. I slowly pulled the hood on my coat over my head. Our clothes were no match for their formal funeral wear.

My father parked the car and we got out. He reached down, grabbed my hand, and held it tight. I dragged my feet and resisted his stride. Finally, my hand slipped free from his. I stuffed it in my pocket. There, I found the red apple. It filled my palm like an oversized baseball. It was cold. I held it tightly.

My father turned around and looked at me, placed his hand over the back of my shoulder, and continued to lead me inside at a slow pace, but it was my pace. My brother followed behind. We walked through the front door and up the center aisle. We passed adults I had never seen before. They turned in our direction. With their elbows, they nudged the person next to them, or tipped their heads awkwardly, at a slant in my direction. I lowered my head and averted my eyes.

My father led us up front to a row of chairs in front of my mother's casket. He sent my brother in first. Then I filled the chair next to him. My father sat next to me in an aisle seat. I didn't want to look but I was sitting near the casket, and for a second, I could make out a darkened bloated profile of a woman. I looked away.

When mourners paid their respects, my father stood up to greet them. Other times he stayed in his seat with his hands supporting his forehead. His eyes welled up with tears.

"We are sorry," I heard again and again from mourners. They shook my father's hand. They patted him on the shoulder. They hugged him.

I was invisible. No one asked how I was or how I felt, or if I was frightened. Then again, I didn't look up when they came to pay their respects. Besides, what do you tell a nine-year-old boy who just lost his mother? *She is in a better place. She is with God now.* Hearing those words would not have made me feel any better. It hurt too much for me to listen to their pity. I was the one who just lost his mother. *What were they sorry for?*

If they had asked how I was feeling, I would have told them that I was worried about a dog. "That on the drive here, we ran over a dog. It was not our fault. The dog ran into the street. He did not see us coming. By the time we saw him, it was too late. After driving over the dog, we did not stop to help. We left him there. We drove away and left him lying in the middle of the road."

If someone had asked what I needed, I would have said that I needed to go back and find that dog. I needed to know that someone told his family where to find him. I needed to explain what happened and that it was not our fault. I knew that it was not our fault, but I needed them to know that we were sorry for leaving him there. That we were on our way to my mother's funeral. I needed them to know that we should have stopped.

But no one asked me how I felt. No one asked what I needed. No one said a word to me. And so, I never looked up.

Near the end of the service, Mrs. Rainer came from behind and placed her hand on my shoulder. She said nothing; she just placed her hand on my shoulder and left it there. When she did, the funeral program fell from my hand and onto the floor. I took in a big breath and nervously let it out. Then she came around front and knelt down before me. Taking my hand in hers, she asked if I wanted to visit my mother one last time before they closed the casket. "I promise to go up with you," she said.

I looked down and slowly shook my head.

"You don't want to see your mother?" she asked.

I shrugged my shoulders. Then after a brief pause, I said, "That can't be my mother. My mother's face was not bloated. My mother's skin was not dark and blotchy. Besides, my mother never sleeps on her back."

Mrs. Rainer slowly nodded in agreement and stayed with me a while longer. Then she lessened her grip on my hand. Finally, she stood up and did what everyone else did. She left, but not before saying, "I am sorry, so very sorry."

15

HER SHOES

The day after the funeral, I walked past my parents' bedroom door. Then I slowly turned around and walked back. This time, I stopped. I peered in. The bed was made, the bed covers were smooth, and the corners neatly tucked. The floor was clean, and the closet doors were closed. No one had slept in that room for several days or nights, not even my father.

I wanted the light entering the room to be warm, to pour through the window in rays of amber and gold, and lift me, and cradle me, and wash me in memory. I wanted the room to smell like my mother, her warm jasmine tea, and her favorite hand cream. I wanted the room to feel the way it used to—like someone I cared for, who cared for me, still lived here.

But it was the middle of January. January in Chicago was cold. And the sky was gray; the light was harsh. And it plunged through the window in shades of metallic gray. The light pushing through the curtains was frigid, and empty, and revealed that everything that belonged to my mother, and reminded me of her, was gone.

I walked in and stood in front of her closet. I slid the door open. The closet was empty. Standing there, I imagined how it was once filled with her dresses, and her coats, and her shoes, and my favorite hiding places.

Who took all her clothes? I wondered.

Five days before, I saw my aunts, all four of her sisters, sifting through her dresses. When they were done, they took only one, the muted pink dress. The dress with pleats, the small waist, and the long hem. The dress that smelled like my mother and her favorite perfume.

I'd watch her put on that dress. She'd lift it over her head, slip into it from the bottom and slide the fabric down over her hips. She'd fasten the belt around her waist and look in the mirror, swinging her body from side to side. Then she'd smile, reach down, and hug me so tightly that my body would rise up against hers and my feet would lift from the floor. I knew where that dress was. Her sisters also knew that she loved that dress; that was why they buried her in it.

But what about her gray dress and her green dress, and all of the other dresses? And where was her soft pink sweater? The one I'd lean into when sitting next to her on the couch.

Where were her shoes? The white tennis shoes that she wore when we walked to Lake Michigan to watch the sunrise over the rippling waves. The sand bogged down our pace as we walked over the shore. She held my hand, my arm stretched out between us as I tried to keep up. Before entering the house, she would take off those shoes and shake out the sand. She'd carry them in her hand, and casually walk up the stairs and into the house in her stocking feet. I'd take off my shoes, shake out the sand, and follow her up the stairs.

Who took her sandals, the ones with the gold straps and flat bottoms? She really liked those shoes. She would paint her toenails bright red when she wore those shoes. She'd ditch the socks and rub lotion all over her feet and her ankles and then up her legs as far as she could reach. She had a way of walking in those sandals. It was carefree. Her hips were loose. When she walked, the bottom of those sandals would flop down and hit the pavement with a slap, and then flop up and hit the soles of her feet with a clap. I expected her to cha-cha or mambo down the sidewalk in those shoes. *Who took her sandals?*

Where are her serious shoes? The black dress shoes? The ones with the pointed toes and tall skinny heels. If I put my feet in those shoes and tried to stand, I would fall sideways into her and she would catch me, and then tell me to put them back in the closet. When she wore those shoes, I knew to fetch her perfume and hand it to her. I would reach in her top dresser drawer and find her pearl necklace and matching earrings. She looked so beautiful with her shoulder-length hair tucked back behind her ears. I knew not to step on those shoes or smear her makeup when she reached down to kiss me goodbye.

I rushed to the dresser. *Where was her perfume?* It was supposed to be here in the glass bottle on the top of her dresser. Her hairbrush and her hand mirror were also missing. I pulled open the top drawer—nothing. Not her pearl necklace, not her slim delicate silver wristwatch, and none of her jewelry. Not even the spare buttons from her coat. Everything was gone. No nylons, no underwear, no pajamas, no loose bobby pins.

How am I going to survive without her?

I knelt down and dropped my body over the edge of the bed. I remembered how I'd whisper her name to wake her up when I could not sleep. She would pull me under the covers, and we both slept until morning.

I lay down on the bed in my usual spot, which was next to her. The place I slept when I was frightened or lonely. The place I slept, when my father worked the midnight shift, to make sure that she was not frightened or lonely, I would tell her.

I would lie next to her and press my back into her belly. So I rounded my back, moving it in the direction where she would have been. She would wrap her body around mine, and I would feel her warmth and her love. So I lifted the covers and placed them over me. She would rest her chin on the top of my head. So I scrunched her pillow and pressed it snuggly against the top of my head. She would wrap her arms around my chest and pull me in so close. So I wrapped my arms around my chest as tight as I could.

But it wasn't the same. I did not feel warm. I did not feel protected. I felt alone. She was never coming back. Each time I said it, I trembled. She was never coming back—never coming back.

I lay there for a long while. Then I turned on my side and stared into the empty closet. I slowly drew up my knees, transforming my body into a huge question mark. *Who would have taken all of her things out of my life as if she had never existed, and as if I did not want to remember?*

PART II

WITHOUT
HER

16

THE MONKEY AND THE VETERINARIAN

At thirty-six, my father was young enough to walk away from his current life and build a new one. If he had, he would have avoided the neighbors' gossip about my parents' failing marriage, their drinking, and their fighting. If he had, he would have escaped the neighbors' inquisitive stares and roundabout conversations trying to unearth the specifics of my mother's death. They thought that they were clever, but I saw through their falsehearted sympathy. They'd say, "I had no idea how much trouble Betty was in," pause and wait for my father to fill in the details. I could hear what they were thinking before they ever asked. *Was she drunk? Did she drink herself to death? Was she insane? Did you kill her?* Wanting-to-know is human nature, but bleeding it out of my distraught father was heartless.

If my father walked away from his current situation, he would have avoided the relentless interrogation from the in-laws. *What did you do to my daughter? How could she die like that? Why didn't you take her to the hospital sooner?* No matter how thoroughly he explained the circumstances, no answer was sufficient to take away my grandparents' pain and their suspicion of my father's involvement.

I could not blame them for thinking the way they did. They lost their daughter. They needed answers to put their life back together. They needed to know that they did everything possible to prevent their daughter's death.

If my father walked out on his current life, he would have surrendered the burden of raising my brother and me. We needed him now more than ever. We needed him to be our father and our mother. But in the immediate aftermath of my mother's death, my father was vulnerable, and we knew it. Bringing up our mother's death would drop him to his knees. And when we were hurting, that is exactly what we did. We would blame him and convince him that it was all his fault.

I knew what my father was thinking. I knew what he was capable of. I knew because I watched him. If he left the house without me, I'd rush to the living room window and peer through a crack I made between the curtain and window frame. I watched him open the door to our blue station wagon, sit behind the wheel, start the engine, and shift out of park only to turn off the ignition, lower his forehead to the top of the steering wheel, and sob. I watched the time he pulled away from the curb only to drive around the block, return home, park the car, and sit there for hours talking to himself before coming back into the house.

I knew what he was capable of the afternoon my brother and I got into a fight with each other. My brother punched me square in the middle of my chest. He hit me so hard that I fell backward and lost my balance. After standing up, I punched him back. He grabbed me around the neck, threw me to the floor, and pummeled into my stomach with his fists.

Before my mother died, my father would have broken it up. He would have shouted at us to stop. But this time was different. He did not shout at us. He did not pull us apart. Instead, he solemnly warned us.

"If you boys don't stop, I am going to have to give you both away."

His words gutted me. I let go of my grip from around my brother's waist. My brother released his clutch from around my neck and pushed me to the side as he got off me. I lay there with my back flat against the floor, staring up at the ceiling. My lip was bleeding. My hands pressed against the pain spreading across my chest. Then I silently repeated every word that my father just said because I knew what he was capable of.

I knew that my brother didn't care. He was twelve, getting older, and beginning to assert his independence. I was only nine and had just lost my mother. I could not imagine losing my father too. From then on, I let my brother win. I avoided any confrontation. If he came looking for me, I didn't come home. If he hit me, I held my breath and remembered not to defend myself. When he hit me harder, I closed my eyes and ignored how much it hurt. No matter how often he goaded me, confiscated my money, or destroyed my toys, I let it go. *I had to.*

I knew what my father was capable of, but in the end, he did not do what he seemed to threaten. He did not avoid the neighbors or the in-laws. He answered their questions in a thoughtful and respectful manner, even if it implicated him. He did not abandon us or send us away. He raised my brother and me with the best intentions and his best efforts. We didn't have the cleanest house or newest clothes. Our life was not organized or normal. But our house was always warm, and the refrigerator was always full.

What we lacked was my father's affection. After the funeral, he was distant. After all he had been through, he had nothing left for us. To take care of himself, he kept busy. Too occupied to help with our homework. Too busy to have dinner with us. Too empty to realize that we needed his love. Instead, he worked. When he was not making Wheaties at General Mills, his factory job, he repaired washing machines and dryers for the neighborhood Sears, or worked on the house, or in the yard, or on the car. I wish that he had worked on just being there with us.

To make up for his absence, my father brought home things for us to work on, things to keep us busy. Model airplanes and cars for us to assemble and paint. He brought kites for us to fly in the park. We had puzzles. I had a chemistry set and an erector set. He brought home books for us to read. When I asked for piano lessons, he arranged a teacher.

One evening, he brought home a monkey. Not a large monkey, but a small squirrel monkey. The monkey had dark-brown fur, a tan face, and large dark eyes. I can't imagine where my father found him. We had dogs and cats before, but never a monkey. One of my father's customers must have given him the monkey. I suspected that his client couldn't keep him, or abandoned the monkey, and my father thought that it would be a great opportunity for us. And another thing to keep us busy.

The monkey arrived in a four-foot-square, thick-wire cage with a shelf, water, and food bowls, and a solid pan on the bottom to catch the waste. I thought that the monkey would be more like a dog or a cat. I thought that he would sit on our shoulders like monkeys in the movies, but the monkey was not sociable. When let out of his cage, he was like a wild animal. I say "he," as it was obvious when he swung above us on the curtain rod that the monkey was a boy. He climbed up the curtains and dangled from the curtain rods, looking down at us. Once out, he refused to go back in his cage. We were careful to make sure that he didn't escape out the front door. But when we tried to catch him, he would jump from one curtain rod to another, or to a picture hanging on the wall, or a light fixture in the middle of the ceiling. He toppled over lamps and ran behind the furniture. Only when he darted into our bedroom could we successfully catch him. We closed the door and trapped him. I threw a large sheet over him. He squealed and bit us through the sheet. While he was trapped in the sheet, we wrapped him in a thick towel. Once captured, we held him tight, ran to the living room, and threw him back in his cage. I quickly closed the cage door and locked it.

I felt sorry for the monkey. He was spending more time in his cage than out of it. *He needed to be with other monkeys,* I thought. Every time I walked past, I handed him chunks of bananas or grapes. Sometimes he ate them. Sometimes he threw them back at me. After several weeks, he was socialized enough to let us pet him.

We didn't have the monkey for long. After a month, he was not himself. He slowed down. He was no longer interested in seeing me when I came home from school or when I offered him food. When I passed his cage, he'd look up instead of coming to the front and reaching for me through the wire. Several days later, he looked cold. I saw him tremble. I threw several of my T-shirts in the cage. He used them to make a bed. I put a blanket over his cage to keep him warm. A few days later, the monkey stopped eating. I knew this was a very bad sign. I was familiar with death and the body's fading signs preceding it. Once a bird flew right into our front window, but the window was closed. It made a loud thud as it hit the glass before falling to the ground. I ran outside to help, but when I arrived, its breathing stopped, and its mouth slowly opened. The bird was dead. When Lightning, our cocker spaniel, got old, I watched as he got skinnier and skinnier. I took him to bed with me each night to keep him warm and comfortable. When he stopped eating, my father took him to the veterinarian. Lightning never came home. I knew that no matter what you hoped for or prayed for, once the body lets go, there is no turning it around. But I hoped and prayed anyway. I hoped that our monkey would give it one last try. I hoped that the veterinarian my father contacted could turn things around.

The veterinarian came to our house to help the monkey. When I opened the door to let him in, I was stunned. This man looked so peculiar. In front of me was a Black man with caramel-colored skin and bright reddish sandy hair. *This could not be a dye job,* I thought. The color went down to the roots and invaded his eyebrows. *How odd,* I thought. I stood there with the door open, looking up at him as if he were a Martian. I had seen Black people and white people, and Asians and Native Americans and all sorts of mixtures. However, I had never seen a Black man with tightly curled hair the color of flaming wheat erupting from his scalp into a short Afro. To add to the mystery, his cheeks were covered with large red freckles. He looked like a character out of one of my Dr. Seuss books. However, his eyes were like mine. Large dark-brown eyes. So dark brown you could not distinguish the pupil from the iris, but you could see and feel the warmth in his gaze. Finally, my father stepped behind me and invited him inside. I still could not stop staring. He appeared so alien. I could not figure out what he was made of or where he came from. When he caught me gawking at him, he smiled. I raised my eyebrows and sheepishly grinned back, twisting my mouth to one side.

After introducing himself, he looked over my head at the monkey in the cage behind me. He walked over and peered inside the cage. The monkey sat on the bottom and paid him no mind. He looked at the monkey again. This time he cocked his head slightly to one side and squinted his eyes as if he wanted to know what the monkey was thinking.

As odd as he appeared, I liked the sandy-haired man. He was friendly and cheerful. And the way he approached the monkey was gentle. He did not open the cage and pull out the monkey. He could have, but he did not. Instead, he pulled up a chair and set it down near the monkey's cage. Before sitting, he lifted his finger to his lips, motioning me to be quiet. I knelt on the floor behind the chair, but off to one side. I waited and watched with intense curiosity. Then the sandy-haired man sat down in the chair. He stared into the cage. He waited for the monkey to look up in our direction. And when the monkey did, he began talking to him. At first, his voice was barely above a whisper.

"Hey buddy," he said and then paused before introducing himself to the monkey. "I work at the University Animal Labs," he said with the same soothing intonation. "Most of the monkeys I take care of are quite a bit larger than you and stronger than both of us." He told the monkey that we were worried about him. "I hear you are not feeling well and that you are not eating." He leaned a little bit forward and whispered, "I'd like to help." The monkey blinked several times. Then he asked the monkey, "Can I take a closer look?"

The monkey listened intently, his tiny ears rotating back and forth. His eyes widened. The monkey looked up at the veterinarian and then looked back down at the bottom of his cage.

The veterinarian unlocked the cage door but left it closed. I thought that he was ready to reach in and grab the monkey, but the sandy-haired man did not. I thought that the monkey might *want* to come out, but I knew that he would not. And he did not.

The soft-spoken man with the sandy hair, caramel-colored skin, and red freckles put his hands on the top of his thighs, extended his arms, and leaned back in his chair, all the while conversing with the monkey. He told the monkey what he had for dinner. "I had baked chicken, green peas, and a banana." I did not believe that the veterinarian had eaten a banana for dinner. But hearing the word *banana,* the monkey looked up and blinked again. Then he asked the monkey what the monkey had for dinner.

I wanted to answer for the monkey because I knew that the monkey had not eaten anything all day. But before I could say a word, the veterinarian asked the monkey another question.

"How are you feeling? Did you drink any water today?"

Then I figured it out. The monkey was not going to answer him. And the veterinarian was not expecting an answer. He wanted the monkey to relax. He wanted the monkey to trust him, to relax. And after a while the monkey did. Only then did the veterinarian open the cage door. He still did not reach in and grab the monkey. He showed the monkey his open hand, but never stopped talking to him.

After a few minutes, while still sitting in the chair and conversing with the monkey, he reached inside the cage. The monkey stiffened his body and turned away toward the corner. The veterinarian paused but never stopped speaking. Then he stretched out one finger and lightly rubbed the back of the monkey's head. Next, he lightly rubbed under the monkey's chin. At first, the monkey showed no interest. Then the monkey leaned into the veterinarian's finger. The sandy-haired man with the big brown eyes opened his hand again, offering it to the monkey. The monkey froze again. Then the monkey slowly turned around, reached for his hand, climbed into his palm, and wrapped his tail around his wrist. My eyes widened. Goosebumps rose up on both arms. A shiver went up my back, forcing my shoulders up toward my ears. I was amazed at how gentle the veterinarian was and how accepting the monkey became.

He lifted the monkey up and out of his cage and sat him up on a blanket that I quickly put in the sandy-haired man's lap. With his other hand, the veterinarian removed a stethoscope from his pocket and showed it to the monkey, not dangling it over his head, but lower near the monkey's belly. The sandy-hair man explained what it was, how it works, and what he was going to do with it.

"I am going to listen to your breathing," he told the monkey. He put one of the eartips in his ear, pulled apart the eartubes of the stethoscope, and inserted the other eartip into his other ear. He moved the bell of the stethoscope toward the monkey. The monkey looked up and touched the stethoscope with one of his fingers. After the monkey inspected the stethoscope, the veterinarian lowered the bell to the monkey's chest and listened. The monkey did not object. In fact, the monkey let his arm dangle away from his chest, permitting easy access for the veterinarian. After listening to one side of the monkey's chest, the veterinarian listened to the other.

The sandy-haired man was patient. His movements were slow. After listening to the monkey's chest, the sandy-haired man lightly stroked the monkey's lip. Then he lifted one side to look at the color of the monkey's gums. Then he lightly pressed over the monkey's abdomen. The monkey took in a deep breath. I noticed the effort it took for the monkey to fill his lungs and, when letting the air out, how the monkey's whole body collapsed inward, also with effort. I watched, concentrating to understand what it all meant, but I knew it meant something in the monkey's breathing was not normal. Before long, the monkey looked tired. The monkey's eyes half-closed.

I had so many questions for the veterinarian but kept quiet. I was not sure that I wanted to know the answers to my questions.

The veterinarian asked me to reach inside his left coat pocket and remove a small bottle. "You will also find a syringe," he said.

"Is this it?" I said.

He nodded. "Shake the bottle to mix it."

I shook the vial. It looked like the antibiotic shot I got the time I had a painful ear infection.

He asked me to turn the bottle upside down. Then with his free hand, he removed the cap on the syringe and inserted the needle that was attached to the syringe into the rubber stopper on the bottle. He pulled back on the plunger and filled the syringe halfway. Then he removed the needle from the bottle by pulling the syringe downward. He lightly stroked the monkey's side before tenting the skin and inserting the needle. When he pushed on the plunger, the liquid in the syringe went under the monkey's skin. When the monkey did not flinch or squeal, I knew the monkey was very sick. When I was sick, I begged the doctor not to give me a shot. But the nurse held me while the doctor dropped my pants and injected medication into my butt. When the needle went in, I screamed. My mother reassured me that it was necessary, but it hurt just the same. When the monkey got his injection, I whispered to the monkey that it was necessary. But when the monkey didn't complain, I knew that he had given up. The veterinarian loaded his stethoscope, the syringe, and the bottle of medication back in his pockets.

The veterinarian was hopeful when he first examined the monkey. Several times, he nodded in my direction. But, when he was finished, his smile became more serious and less cheerful.

"I cannot make any promises," he told my father. He looked down at me, half-smiled, closed both his eyes and opened them quickly, blinking several times. I pushed my lower lip out in resignation. My father walked him to the door. Before leaving, the veterinarian patted my father on the shoulder. That was the only time that I saw the sandy-haired man with large red freckles and big brown eyes. He had no reason to come back. When I checked the cage in the morning, the monkey was wrapped in one of my old T-shirts that I had given him. I approached the cage, I softly called out his name, "Hey Monkey," but he did not move. Then I softly whistled. Still no movement. I reached in and softly stroked the fur over the back of his neck. His body was stiff. The monkey was dead. And I was crushed. As I look back, the monkey likely had pneumonia or heart failure. Or maybe a broken heart from not being with other monkeys.

The monkey's death was not unexpected; he had been declining for almost a week. What was unexpected were the overwhelming feelings I had after meeting the sandy-haired man with large red freckles and big brown eyes. I was captivated by his compassion and his empathy. He was so gentle with the monkey. I was amazed at his generosity. He gave up his time to let the monkey relax and accept him. I was awed by his ability to communicate with the monkey and gain the monkey's trust. In return, I saw how appreciative the monkey was. I was also humbled by the veterinarian's willingness to let me help. While caring for the monkey, I thought about the dog our car hit on the way to my mother's funeral. I thought about how much that dog would have benefited from someone as caring as the sandy-haired man. With that in mind, it was clear what I had to do. I wanted to be just like the sandy-haired man with large red freckles and kind brown eyes. I wanted to be a veterinarian.

The monkey's life had not been saved, but mine was possibly, if not saved, directed. If I could prevent pain and suffering and death, even sometimes, wouldn't that rescue me, help me heal? The way to do that, I saw right away, was through showing kindness.

17

SCHOOL

I returned to school without the anxiety and urgency of having to rush home. Without my mother, there was no one to rush home to, no one to clean up, no one to put to bed. There were no liquor bottles to hide, no smell of booze to wash from her mouth, and no one to lie for to my father. I had been wired to fix what was wrong with us. As I think back, maybe I was taught or manipulated to cover up the truths about my mother. Either way, without my mother and without her destructive behaviors to conceal or clean up, I was unsure of my role. I no longer had a job to do. But I needed one. I needed to feel loved. And so I latched onto the next possibility.

When I was not at school, I was with my father. I went on service calls with him. I helped him fix the house. I put away the tools and collected up the nails and screws when the job was done. I kept the house clean.

I did my best at school for him. But that was not enough. In high school, I performed at the top of my class in math and science, but I couldn't seem to earn high marks in English. I kept telling myself this was what was lacking, and if I ever could excel in English, he would be proud of me.

Finally, after three years of trying harder, I came home with a report card with all As, even in English! Reading was an escape for me. I could hardly wait to show my father.

"Here you go, Dad," I said as I passed my report card to him with the page showing my grades. He was sitting at the dining room table going through his mail. I went to the opposite side of the table to face him. I waited.

"Where do I sign?" he said without looking up from his mail.

I took a step back, not only in distance but also in time. I tried to remember the father who lovingly cared for me. I tried to remember the father who when he returned from work each day would open his arms to catch me as I ran toward him because he was so happy to see me. He would lift me and carry me on his back. I tried to remember the father who had infinite patience when he taught me to sink a hole and drive a nail. I tried to remember the father who taught me to fly a kite and enjoyed water fights with the garden hose on hot summer afternoons. I tried to remember the father who would kiss me good night before bed, and I would shy away because his mustache tickled. And I tried to remember the father who would carry me in after returning home from the drive-in movies in the summer and watch me fall asleep while he marveled at the astonishment that he made me, that I was a part of him and would always be.

I extended my hand and pointed to the blank line on the bottom of the page where he needed to sign. Then I reached in my shirt pocket and handed him my pen while wondering where was the father I once knew and loved, and thought that he loved me.

18

THE NEIGHBOR BOY

When my parents battled, I thought that my brother was immune to their bickering. During their squabbles, Gary remained quiet and detached. I thought that he had acquired a resiliency and an understanding that I lacked, but I was wrong.

Months after my mother's death, my brother, now thirteen, and I, ten, were home alone. I was eating dinner and finishing my homework at the dining room table. Without warning, my brother grabbed the back of my collar and at the same time kicked my feet forward and out from under me. My head fell backward as I hit the floor. My eyes swept up from the table to the ceiling as I watched the world spin in the wrong direction. He was not done with me. He grabbed my collar and pressed my throat. It was difficult for me to breathe. He dragged me to the front door and shoved me outside. As he pushed me out, I tripped and fell. The lower half of my body landed inside the doorframe. He kicked my feet and legs until every part of me was outside. Then he slammed the door shut and locked it. It was cold outside. There was no time to grab my coat. Besides, he would not have allowed it.

These unprovoked attacks were reminiscent of my father's attacks on my mother. My brother had an unpredictable mean streak, a trigger that went off in his head without warning. And tonight, I was the target. I was safer outside than in the house.

I began to shiver. I pounded on the door with my fists and pleaded with him to let me in. He opened the door with only enough room to throw my schoolwork out and into the wind. My schoolbooks fell from his hands and hit the porch floor. My papers flew up in the air like a flock of birds set free. The door slammed shut. I turned around.

In the distance, my papers flew on the frigid wind and tumbled over the snow.

The tall lanky teenager with caramel skin and sandy-brown hair who lived across the street saw what happened. He came over to help. He chased my loose papers as they blew down the street. He trapped them under his shoe and waited for me to rush behind, reach down, and grab them. We looked foolish chasing papers, but together, we retrieved them all.

He removed his jacket and handed it to me.

"Here, put this on," he said.

The sleeves were long and covered my hands. I balled my fists up inside the cuffs to keep them warm.

I had nowhere to go. He took me home with him. We ate sandwiches in his kitchen. In slow motion, he reenacted what our bodies did chasing papers down the street. Reaching in the air to catch imaginary sheets of my homework, he grabbed my nose and squeezed it. We both laughed.

After eating, he took me upstairs to his room. The room was small with a narrow window, a single twin bed, and a wooden desk against the wall. Unlike my room, there were no plastic models of cars in various stages of assembly. My life was messy. His room was neat and organized.

The light entering through the window was fading. He said that I could rest until my father came home. I lay down. He went back downstairs to clean the dishes in the kitchen. When he returned, he climbed the stairs quietly.

I was lying on my back with my head on his pillow and my eyes closed. He kneeled on the floor next to me. He reached over and rested his hand on my belly. He slowly unbuttoned the bottom of my shirt. He slid his index finger inside my belly button and slowly skated around its rim. His touch was soft. I counted each circle he made. *One, two, three, four.*

He slowly moved his finger outside my navel. His circles grew larger. Instead of using one finger, he now used two. I kept counting.

Twenty-two, twenty-three, twenty-four. His hand slipped below the waist of my pants.

"*Uh.*" I breathed in sharply and held it. I tensed my abdomen. I opened my eyes and stared straight up at the white ceiling. I remained perfectly still and disappeared between its fine cracks and speckled texture until it was over.

From then on, I never walked on that side of the street where his house was. If I saw him out on his porch or in his front yard, I never looked in that direction. One day, he waved at me and I pretended to not see him. I just kept walking. I didn't tell my father either. I should have, but I didn't want to relive any part of it, even the retelling. I didn't know if my father would blame me for something I had no control over.

19

———

DOROTHY

"Don't buck me." Those were the words Dorothy shouted as she shoved me down the basement stairs. At the same time, she had collected my shirts from my closet and threw them down the stairs after me. With the door closed, and the latch fastened, I would remain locked in the basement for the rest of the night until my father came home.

Dorothy had arrived one year after my mother's death. It was December 1967. My father said he went out drinking, picked her up at a bar, and brought her home. I am not sure that is true. What is true is that my father went out one evening, and when he returned, she walked in the door with him and lived with us for the next three months.

Dorothy was five feet six, slender, dark-skinned, with tightly curled brown hair. I am not sure what my father saw in her, but he catered to her. It was a shock for me to come home from school and see an aluminum Christmas tree. A rotating color wheel on the floor lit up the tree like a neon sign, first blue, then green, then orange, and finally red, changing color every fifteen seconds. It was nothing like the real Christmas trees with our traditional ornaments that we had when my mother was alive. This woman who did not work was getting my father to buy garish unnecessary things when my brother and I had a hard time convincing him to buy what was essential for us.

The incident happened when I came home from school and saw Dorothy in the bedroom I shared with my brother. Even before my mother died, I used to do my own laundry. We had a washing machine and dryer in the basement. Instead of folding my shirts and storing them in drawers, I hung them from hangers in the closet. Dorothy was angry because my shirts were wrinkled. Previously she had asked me to iron them, but I never ironed my shirts. I didn't mind going to school in wrinkled shirts. She grabbed them and began tossing them down the basement stairs while screaming at me that she told me to iron them. When I said that I was not going to iron them, she said, "Don't buck me," and locked me in the basement. Why should she even care how wrinkled my shirts were? She saw me as defiant. When I complained to my father, he sided with her. As much as I loved my father, I no longer felt safe, and at eleven years old, I moved out.

The neighborhood where we lived was great for kids. I felt welcome in most houses on my block. On my side of the street, there were the Despeoles and the Galvins. Across the street were the Bells, the Grahams, and the Browns.

The Galvins were particularly friendly to Gary and me. They lived two houses down the street in a large two-story blue frame house. My brother and I often played with their two boys, Kenny and Porky. When I showed up with a brown paper bag full of my clothes and schoolbooks the day after Dorothy locked me in the basement, they were happy to have me.

Ora Lee lived on the first floor. We called her MaDear, which was short for Mother Dearest. She would be my new grandmother. She was older than the rest of the grownups on the street, probably in her fifties at the time. She never drove a car and had to get up around five in the morning to take the bus to work. I'd meet her walking home at the end of her day. She was the one who was more of a disciplinarian. She'd tell us to slow down and stop running through the house. She was also the kindest. She'd sit us kids down next to her and pat us on the knee and we'd watch TV together. When she passed through downtown Chicago on the way home from work, she'd pick up Fannie May Turtles, pecan caramel clusters covered in milk chocolate. She'd dole them out. Not only were they more expensive than beef, but they were so delicious, and one was never enough.

On the second floor lived her daughter, Jessie, the mother of Kenny, Porky, and Diane. She never talked about Mr. Galvin, who was no longer in the picture, and I never asked. Jessie was very attractive, with her medium-brown complexion and shoulder-length hair, and she knew it. She had several male suitors who came by often. I was surprised that none of them collided with one another. At times I thought that she drank too much, but I worried about that more than anyone else, since I saw what happened to my mother. But it never stopped her from working. She worked for the post office during the week and had a part-time beauty parlor in the enclosed back porch on her apartment level. What I liked most about Jessie is that she just seemed to enjoy life. She and her friends would get together, drink, smoke cigarettes, and hoot with laughter. I admired and envied how happy she was.

Holidays at their house were the best. They made a feast with turkey and real macaroni and cheese, nothing from a box. They had chitlins, collard greens, and cornbread made in a heavy black cast-iron skillet. The sweet potato pies were made from scratch and topped with toasted marshmallows. The table was set by 1:00 p.m. and was so full of food that you grabbed a plate and sat down on the couch to eat. Everyone was welcome—neighbors, kids, visiting relatives. The eating did not stop until well past 10:00 p.m. Regular dinners were just as good, with fried chicken, spaghetti, and soda pop, or barbecued ribs and hamburgers. Living with them ensured that I was going to put some meat on my skinny bones.

I stayed with the Galvins for a month. I stayed until the day I walked past my house on the way to school and saw the front window boarded up. Dorothy was gone, but not until she and my father had a fight. I guess that she was too much to handle for any of us. My father said that she cornered him with a knife and he had to jump through the front window to save his life. Good thing we lived on the first floor.

MaDear, Jessie, and her children were my second family. I spent the night whenever I wanted to and whenever I needed to. When they went on vacations, they took me along. Dinner was always an open invitation. I showed my appreciation by clearing the table and washing the dishes or running errands, and telling them how much

I cherished their kindness. For many of my graduations, when my father was always absent, Ora Lee and Jessie were the only family members in the audience cheering me on. We maintain that sense of family today. We kids call one another cousin, and Kenny's daughters affectionately call me Uncle Jody.

20

—

THELMA

Early on, I came to realize that my father needed companionship and I needed a mother. We needed two different things from the same person, and most of the time, it did not work out that way.

After Dorothy, there was Vivian. Vivian had so much going for her, a beautiful house, a well-paying job as a hospital administrator, and she would not be an easy catch. She liked my father, but she was going places and had been in situations that my father didn't quite fit in. She was too sophisticated for a factory worker. They remained good friends and in each other's lives, but nothing more materialized.

Then there was Ethel, a beautiful woman with a good caring heart. She was a dental hygienist, and for the first time, I was visiting a dentist regularly, instead of only when I had a toothache. She and her two boys lived with us for three years. When I saw the relationship deteriorating, I was sad.

There were a few others. But they came and went so quickly that I do not remember their names.

Years later, when I was fifteen and running late for school, I knocked on my father's bedroom door while turning the knob and pushing open the door. I needed bus fare and lunch money. Instead, I got a front-row view of my father in bed having sex with Thelma. At the time, I didn't know her name. I quickly closed the door and managed with the little money I had to get to school and back. By the time I came home that afternoon, both were gone. That was to be expected, since that week my father was working the second shift.

I would finally meet Thelma the following weekend. She lived with two of her sisters in the Washington Heights neighborhood on the far south side of Chicago. All the houses in the neighborhood were small tan-brick bungalows built in the 1960s. All of them had brick stairs leading to the front door and, on the other side, a large living room window with a view of the street. We climbed the front steps to ring the doorbell, but before we leaned into it, Thelma opened the door to greet us.

Thelma's skin was a dark shade of chocolate, and she had dark-auburn hair. Her face possessed a slight layer of fat beneath her complexion that smoothed out any harsh angular features. Her complexion and full lips accentuated a bright white smile with perfect teeth. At five and a half feet tall, she fit neatly under my father's arm. She was not fat, but she also was not thin. She looked the same age as my father, early forties. She put her arms around me and pulled me into the house, dumping me into the living room as if we had been best friends for many years. That's when I saw her sister, Wardine, sitting on the couch with her arms folded in front of her.

Wardine is an old German name meaning "guardian," and it fit her perfectly. She didn't get up to greet us. She scowled with disappointment and disapproval. She knew what I did not. We were not there to visit. Thelma grabbed a few changes of clothes and some necessities from the bathroom, headed out the front door, and got in our car. Thelma was coming home with us.

Of the women my father dated, I liked Thelma the most. She was kind and encouraging. Her friendliness was open and unconditional.

Thelma was not a morning person. She worked the second shift, 3:00 p.m. to 11:30 p.m., as a nurse at the nearby University of Chicago hospitals. She also worked a shorter week, Thursday to Monday.

Within a month of moving in, Thelma called home one Saturday. I picked up the phone and said hello.

"Is your father at home?" she asked. "I need a favor."

"Dad's out on a service call," I told her. "Is there anything that I can do?"

Without a pause, Thelma said, "Yes."

Thelma told me that she was taking care of a woman with

esophageal cancer. "Her esophagus is raw and painful after the radiation treatment. I'm feeding her through a stomach feeding tube coming out the side of her abdomen because she should not take anything orally, including water. The woman will not stop asking me for chocolate. What should I do?"

I was thinking that the woman should have her chocolate. If I had a bad disease, all I would want is vanilla ice cream. All that I could eat.

Then Thelma told me her plan: "Why not put the chocolate through the feeding tube?" Thelma snickered in the phone and whispered, "I hope the lady is not listening. I want to surprise her. Jody, I need you to go to the store and buy a bag of Hershey's Kisses. Can you do that for me?"

I got on my bike, made a stop at the grocery store, and delivered the goods to the main entrance of the hospital. Thelma came down and greeted me with an appreciative hug before taking the bag of chocolates and disappearing down the hallway.

When Thelma came home that evening, I asked, "How did it go?"

First, she told me that she didn't tell the doctors anything about her plan. "I unwrapped a couple of Hershey Kisses for myself and put the rest in a blender. I added warm water. Turned on the switch and ground it into a slurry. I scooped a small amount out with a tongue depressor to taste. The batch was too thick. I could hardly suck it up into the syringe. I added more water and voilà, a smooth creamy chocolate treat. I filled a syringe. Then I pumped the chocolate through her feeding tube. The woman rubbed her belly, smacked her lips, and purred mmm mmm good. The lady and I just laughed and laughed because we knew that she could not taste any of it."

I began to laugh and shake my head at the same time as Thelma finished the story. Thelma had many good qualities, but she was not a good cook. I was surprised to hear how well she did with a blender. It was not until Thelma came to live with us that I heard about Spam. Spam was this canned meatloaf of pork, potato starch, and salt. It was difficult to look at and even more horrible to taste. Sometimes she would eat it fresh out of the can, and other times sliced and fried. It didn't matter; no one liked it but Thelma.

Thelma did change our house in a different way. After my mother died, our father stopped smoking and drinking and became quite the health nut. He was buying fruit by the case and telling us to eat less red meat. After my mother died, we rarely ate desserts or other sweet treats. Thelma, on the other hand, must have never had a meal without following it up with something sweet. Sometimes Thelma would have the sweet stuff before the meal. On the days that Thelma didn't work and my father did, I would catch her sitting up in bed reading or watching TV. She would pat the bed and invite me up. Then she would pull out her hidden stash of donuts from under the bed. She needed a partner in crime, since my father didn't approve. Little did I know that I was not just her partner in crime, I was the criminal. When my father found her stash of goodies, instead of confessing, she told him that they were mine. For many months, I had no idea that I was her scapegoat until my father cornered me in the backyard and asked why I was eating such terrible unhealthy food. I marched into the house and confronted Thelma. Without an inkling of remorse, she turned it around back on me. She made me feel guilty for not covering for her. She would tell me how much she had done for me and why would I not do this one little thing for her. I gave up. I could not win with either of them.

21

COLLEGE

After high school, I attended Northwestern University in Evanston, Illinois. My transition to college was difficult. Emotionally, I was not ready to leave home. I was nothing more than a hurt child wanting his father's love and approval. All the other college students were celebrating their independence, rejoicing in their freedom from parental oversight. Now that I was miles away from home, I felt isolated. And because my father never phoned to check in on me, I felt abandoned.

I tried to study, but I kept wondering why? Who cares if I live or die, I often thought. Some days, I missed my morning classes because I didn't have the inclination to get out of bed when I thought that I might not live long anyway. Academically, I was not failing, but it was close. I was certainly no better than average. I was a disappointment to myself, which meant that I would be a disappointment to my father. Initially, I didn't want to leave home. Now that I was struggling, I didn't know how to go back. But I had no choice. During Christmas break, the dormitory would close.

I boarded the commuter train from Evanston to downtown Chicago. Looking out the window, I saw sparks from the metal wheels passing over the steel rails, shooting flares of light against the sides of the train cars.

As all the trains come in from the outer ring of cities, some remain elevated while others dive underground. The line that I was riding submerged below the city streets as it approached downtown. When the train stopped at Jackson Street, I got off, took the escalator up, and boarded the number 6 Jeffery express bus going south to Hyde

Park. I got off at Forty-Seventh Street and Lake Park and walked the rest of the way home.

When I arrived, the lights were out. No one was home. I used my key to get in.

I walked past the kitchen. Dirty dishes filled the sink. I was the family dishwasher. It was not always that way. My brother and I were to take turns each week. But he rarely completed the chore. He would let dishes pile up, especially near the end of the week when the chore passed over to me, leaving me with more than my share. So when I came home from college and saw a sink full of dirty dishes, it felt familiar. I had work to do.

I took off my backpack and my coat and placed them on the floor. I cleared the dishes from the sink, putting them in order of how I would wash them. I was good at putting things in order. Order somehow calmed me, having grown up in extreme chaos. With the hot water running, I placed the stopper in the drain and squirted in a few jets of liquid dish detergent. The soap made everything slippery. I took care of the big things first, the bowls, the plates, and the pans. I rinsed them and set them on the rack to dry. I picked up a drinking glass and filled it with soapy water, then poured the water back out. The caked-on globs on the inside looked like someone scrambled eggs in it and then set it aside and it dried. I grabbed a small dishcloth out of the soapy water and stuffed it inside the glass. I pushed my hand down into the glass. I rotated my hand clockwise and then rotated it back. When I rotated it back, the glass cracked. The dishwater turned pink. I lifted my hand. A slice of my flesh dangled from the back of my hand over my index finger. Blood oozing up from the wound dripped from my fingertip and rippled through the network of interlacing suds floating on top.

I don't know what came over me, but I began searching for the broken piece of glass, the one that cut me. I can't explain how I felt. I searched the bottom of the sink until I found it. It was more a reaction than a thought. I pushed the sharp end of the glass into my left wrist. The skin indented and then the blood welled up over my wrist.

At first, it didn't hurt. The pain of losing my mother and being alone was worse than any cut I could make. But I wanted my father to notice how much pain I was in. I wanted him to know that I needed him. I held my breath and pushed the glass deeper, opening the wound until blood gushed out.

I heard the front door open. Only then did the pain rise up to the top of my head so intensely that I wanted to scream. But I didn't. I knew better. My father was not going to love me because I hurt myself, I realized.

I quickly emptied the sink and rinsed away the blood. I grabbed a towel, wrapped it around my hand and another towel around my wrist. I ran to the bathroom and cleaned myself up. I hid my wounds under a few bandages and a whole lot of shame.

I never told anyone. Not how I felt. Not that I hurt myself.

I returned to college as soon as the dormitory reopened. The accidental wound on the back of my right hand and the self-inflicted wound on my left wrist would heal. *But would I?*

In college, another realization emerged. Cecilia, a beautiful woman, invited me to her dormitory room on a Friday night. Her caramel-colored complexion was smooth and unblemished. Her dark-auburn shoulder-length hair was soft and supple. I was a sophomore and she was a freshman. When I arrived, she opened the door, smelling like a bouquet of flowers.

The dormitory rooms were square boxes constructed from concrete cinder blocks. The outline of the cinder blocks was a prominent feature of dormitory walls. Each room housed two people. A closet, a twin bed, and a desk in a line leading to a large window. The other side was a perfect match. Hers was no different, but tonight she was alone.

She invited me in. I sat on the edge of her bed. I am not sure what I was expecting, but without asking, she laid her upper torso across my lap and closed her eyes. I was startled, not by her actions but mine. My arms fell to my sides and I froze. I was frightened.

Ever since my mother died, I no longer wanted to be touched that way or touch someone else. I could not help but remember that love only comes with loss. Touching was okay as long as it was not romantic or personal. Touch was only welcomed if I had little to lose. And there was something else. I liked looking at guys more than girls. I liked watching the male cheerleaders during the football games. I got excited at their strength and the way they held hands with the other men to support the women cheerleaders during formations and stunts. However, after staring for a minute, I would shake my head and murmur not for me. I blamed my mother for probably being drunk when she was pregnant with me. Of course, I didn't know if she was drunk. I also blamed my father for withholding his affection when I needed it the most. I didn't know what to feel. I thought that once I got better, I would be normal. I wanted a family and to be a father. However, feeling the way I did about being touched and by whom, maybe I should have a different plan for the future. I had to decide if I was going to be happy or if I wanted my father to be proud of me. For now, I chose the latter.

PART III

GRACE

22

LEAVING HOME

I knew what I wanted to do with my life. I knew how I was going to finally get my father's love and approval. Near the end of college, I applied to three veterinary schools. All three rejected me. My grades weren't good enough. My standardized test scores weren't high enough. My professional-related experience wasn't sufficient. I returned home a failure. I worked as an electron microscopist evaluating the microanatomy of diseased hearts at the University of Chicago, which was a short walk from home. After correcting my deficiencies, I reapplied the following year. Tuskegee, one of America's historically Black universities, accepted me. I was thrilled, but I had never lived in the South before, and in my mind, Alabama was the Deep South.

When I boarded the airplane in Chicago, I had two suitcases, one with my books and the other with my clothes, and a small amount of cash that I saved for the journey. The first stop was Atlanta, Georgia. We landed on time. I walked through the terminal for an hour before catching my flight to Alabama. Instead of boarding by a jetway, we were led down a staircase to the tarmac. When the crew opened the door leading out, I heard the man in front of me say, "Jesus, this is hot."

In the distance, our airplane seemed to undulate, a mirage, as hot air rose from the pavement and mingled with cooler air above it.

"Good or bad, change is coming," said the same man in front of me.

I felt it too. The air—hot, heavy, and thick with moisture—flowed down my lungs like molasses. On the short walk to the plane, sweat simmered up from beneath my skin and pooled in the middle of my back. My blue shirt quickly became a mosaic of wet and dry splotches. The heat was eating me alive.

Our plane looked like a large crop duster, a two-engine, four-seater with room for luggage in the back. A fierce red stripe whipped its way across the side of the white fuselage from the nose to the tail in a wavy pattern indicative of speed and nimbleness.

We approached on the right. A small two-step, metal staircase provided easy entry. The other two passengers boarded first. I sat up front with the pilot. The flight started out smooth. The sun was high, and there was hardly a cloud in the sky. But that didn't last. As we flew west, the sky turned ominously gray, and billowing clouds encircled our plane. I saw flashes of lightning ignite the clouds in the distance. Then came the rain. It pelted the windshield with machine-gun precision. A sudden flash of lightning closer to us jolted the plane.

The pilot remained calm as the plane dipped, veered up, and dipped again. Even with the safety belt fastened tightly around my waist, I firmly held on to the bottom of my seat to steady myself.

Steady myself? I didn't do that so well this morning before leaving home and boarding this plane. I had no idea that my father and I would part in such silence. When I got out of bed, my father was already awake. We both knew that I was leaving for Alabama. But there was no father-son talk. That talk about his overarching view of the world and where I fit in. How do you tell your twenty-two-year-old son, who thinks he knows the world, your overarching view? How do you tell your twenty-two-year-old son, who has been more of a parent to himself than his father, any of your views? We both knew what we needed. And if it hadn't happened in twenty-two years, it wasn't likely to happen now.

Instead, he handed me a list of fifteen chores. "Dad," I scowled with reservation, "I have to leave home by noon to catch my flight." Then I acquiesced and gave my more appropriate response. I nodded. "Okay, I will do what I can."

I wasn't sure if this list was his way of telling me not to go, or he would miss me, or that he needed me. I wasn't sure if he really needed my help. I took it at face value, and I did what I could. *At least he didn't have painting on the list,* I thought. I pulled out the handcart to move the large garbage drums. They were full of trash from us clearing out the basement the previous night. That was yesterday's list. I wheeled them into the alley for the garbage collector. Then I moved the large flowerpots up front and spaced them evenly along the driveway. Next, I dug a hole in the backyard to bury the compost. My father was good to the earth even before being good to the earth was popular. We stored vegetable waste in an old white plastic five-gallon paint container. When it was full, we buried the slop. It smelled horrible, worse than rotten food. But the vegetables he planted around the compost were the best on the block. Good can come from rotten; it just depends on how you cultivate it.

Then he asked me to help carry the table saw from the garage into the backyard. "There are a few boards on the fence that need replacing," he said.

The only problem with that fence was that it was taller than city code allowed. We didn't like neighbors looking in our backyard. And we did not like seeing our neighbors. So my father had built the fence six feet tall, with the slats touching one another.

I held the wood steady while he carefully positioned a new slat on the table saw. When I was a little boy, I helped by holding the board over my head. Now, we were the same height, the same weight, the same brown eyes, and we had the same family history. When I looked across the saw at my father, I looked straight into his eyes. He was staring down at the wood, adjusting its position with the blade of the saw. I hoped that he would look up at me. I wanted to complete that thread woven together between a father and son that words cannot completely convey, especially as I was leaving home soon and wasn't sure if I would ever live at home again. In the middle of my hopeful stare, sawdust flew up in the air between us as he started the saw and pushed the wood against the whirring blade.

"A perfect cut," he remarked. Together, we cut three more slats, the blade screaming as it sliced through the wood and whistling when the cut was complete. The fresh smell of cut cedar did its best to ease my apprehensions. "We're done," he said. My father went into the garage, and when he came out, he had screws and a level in one hand, and a can of brown paint and a paintbrush in the other. I laughed because I knew what was coming, and it was not on the list.

"I'll fix the broken sections while you touch up the fence before you go," he said.

"Touch up" was a euphemism for painting the entire fence. I wasn't sure that I had time to paint the entire fence. I started at the back, making sure that the new slats got a protective coating of primer. When I was done painting, I looked up at my father and said, "Dad, I need to go. I need to clean myself up and there are still a few things that I need to pack."

He stopped what he was doing and slowly walked toward me. He was close enough to hug me. But instead, he reached in his pocket and pulled out a handful of money, mostly fifty- and one-hundred-dollar bills. It looked like a lot of money.

"Here, take it," he said. And offered it up to me.

My hands, splattered with paint, and free of expectation, reached for the money. But, in midreach, I stopped. I had a new skin.

"Dad, we talked about this," I said. "I think that I can do this by myself. You paid for college and it was expensive. I think that I can pay for vet school."

"Take the money in case of an emergency," he said.

"I can't, Dad, you've already sacrificed so much."

He took a long look at me one last time. Then motioned the money toward me again. This time I didn't reach for it. This time he didn't utter a word. This time he put his hands back in his pockets and the money went back in too. And maybe with it, the words he wanted to say and the words I needed to hear. He turned away and walked to the back of the yard.

When I came out with my two suitcases to say goodbye, I couldn't find him. He had planned to drive me to the airport.

I figured it out. I was on my own. Just what I asked for. I walked to the corner and waited for the bus.

I could have handled that better, I thought. Parents are wired to take care of their children. I am not sure if it's instinct, or genetics, or their investment in their old age. I should have taken the money. Offering a gift and being refused was more hurtful than if I took it and never used it. If he thought that I was rejecting him, that was not my intention. But when I needed his love the most, he withheld it. When I needed his approval, he ignored me or corrected me. When I needed his arms to hold and protect me, he told me to get rid of the tears and don't you dare cry. I thought he was toughening me up, preparing me for the world. I thought he wanted me to be independent. To only accept what I've earned, and no more.

What if I really need this money? What if I ask for money in the future and he reminds me how he gave me the chance and I said no? I had no idea where I was going to live, or how much it would cost to finish school. I was on shaky ground with or without his money, with or without his approval, with or without his love. Throughout most of my life, I felt as if I were on my own. What I didn't recognize at the time was how much I was like him. I withheld my love when he needed it the most.

After twenty minutes of precarious flying, the pilot turned his head toward us and announced, "We'll be landing in about fifteen minutes; make sure your seat belts are fastened tight."

My first thought, great, I can't wait to get out of this mess. My second thought, in this torrential storm, how in the hell is he going to land this whirligig?

We started our descent. The landing gear locked into position. The wing flaps engaged. The plane accelerated and the nose pitched upward. Without warning, strong turbulence shoved the plane downward a few hundred feet. We fell through the bottom of the clouds. The plane swerved right and then left, and then right again before the pilot was able to take control. I tightened my seat belt.

In the distance, I could see the lights of the airport flashing.

Crack. Crack. Crack. All of a sudden, blinding flashes of lightning bolted from the clouds to the ground, searing a line in the land below us. The earth unzipped before my eyes. Rocks and dirt spewed into the air. When the dust settled, a ditch wide enough to devour a car stretched an eighth of a mile long.

It was more dangerous to land than to keep flying, I thought. The pilot thought differently. He lined up for the runway and took us down. I closed my eyes and tightly gripped the armrests. The plane tossed so many times, I wasn't sure who was in control, the weather or the pilot. Finally, with a massive thud, the wheels hit the runway. The impact drove us deep into our seats. The engine roared and the wing flaps tipped up. The plane slowed to a land speed that the pilot could control. But without warning, the wind shifted, the wheels skidded over the pavement, and the plane veered sideways. The pilot grunted while he firmly negotiated the yoke, fighting our trajectory and reversing our momentum. With the propellers whirring and rain smashing against the windshield, we somehow got back on track and stayed there until he safely steered us to the gate. He cut the engine. The ground crew ran out from under shelter and placed large blocks in front of and behind all the wheels. The way the wind was gusting, I thought that they should cable the wings to the pavement too. Finally, they wheeled the low metal staircase to the passenger side door.

I looked out the window. Murky russet-colored puddles of water were everywhere, even on the runway. The rain was taking its time to percolate through the red clay soil of Alabama.

I let go and breathed. We made it, I whispered. But not before the young man behind me retched up his lunch. When I heard him gagging and coughing, I crouched forward in my seat to avoid the splatter.

He was not the only one who lost something. When I got off the plane to collect my luggage, I was one suitcase short. And those unspeakable parts of my childhood were farther away than they had ever been before.

23

GRACE

It was a short ride to Tuskegee University. This time in a cab. I arrived before 5:00 p.m. and checked into the dorm. Exhausted from the trip, I didn't unpack. I fell across the bed and slept all night and into the next morning. My lost suitcase with my books arrived the next day.

Having lived in a dormitory during college, I was not looking forward to repeating that living arrangement. Maybe if I were younger, I could tolerate cafeteria food or share a small room with a recent high school graduate. But at twenty-two, I needed more privacy and more quiet.

An apartment of my own would be ideal, but I had to be realistic. An apartment and the additional expenses for utilities were a luxury that I could not afford. It would be considerably less if I rented a room in someone's house. I was also looking for a place close to campus. I did not have a car or a bike.

When I met the dean's secretary the day before, she joked with me about my Midwestern innocence and asked if I had culture shock, since this was my first trip to the South. In my best southern dialect, I said, "I expected everyone to speak with a southern drawl, women would wear hoop skirts like Scarlett O'Hara in *Gone with the Wind*, and you Southerners washed your clothes by beating them against a rock in the river."

We both laughed at my whimsical but feigned immaturity. I liked Barbara. She was friendly, and we could joke with each other even though we had just met. Maybe she could help me find a place to live? I explained my situation and what I was looking for.

She said that she was glad I asked. She told me that when she was a student at Tuskegee, she rented a room from Grace Hooks. She lives close. "I will phone right away," she said.

"Hi Miss G, Barbara here, how are you? Earlier you asked me to keep an eye out for a student to rent that second bedroom in your house. Have you found someone yet?"

After a short pause, Barbara winked at me.

"Perfect," Barbara said into the phone.

Then she cupped her hand over the mouthpiece and whispered, "Can you go see her this afternoon?"

I nodded.

"I will send him your way. I think that you will like him. Great talking with you Miss G. Bye for now."

I followed Barbara's directions. It was a twenty-minute walk down the main road through town. The red brick on all the houses reminded me of the red clay that they stood on and the history that Tuskegee University, a historically Black college, was built on. A hundred years ago, in 1881, Booker T. Washington was hired to lead Tuskegee to train African American teachers for the segregated South. When he arrived, there were no buildings, only land, rich red clay. In the neighboring Episcopal church, he taught the students how to work with their heads. And in the fields that would soon become Tuskegee University, he taught them how to work with their hands—how to gather up the red clay and make bricks, how to arrange the bricks into a foundation, and how to build upon that foundation a great school to teach students to be wise and self-reliant.

I had been in Tuskegee for only two days, but I was beginning to feel as if things were going to work out. With the little money I had saved, staying on track would require wise thinking and a few sacrifices. I wouldn't have to gather up red clay and make bricks, but I would have to be frugal with my money. If the rent was reasonable, I wouldn't have to worry much about tuition and books. If the rent was more than what I set aside, I could spend less on food, and use the books in the library. I continued my walk down the main road through town with renewed hope that I was going to finish this and make my father proud.

When I reached Bibb Street, I turned left and went up the road. At the top of the hill, just as Barbara described, was a modest, one-story California bungalow with light green horizontal siding. At the foundation of that bungalow were those familiar red bricks. 1101 Bibb Street. It matched the address on the note that Barbara gave me. The front of the house had a large covered porch and a wrought iron railing. The roof was pitched at multiple sections to direct rainwater away from the house. The driveway on the side didn't lead to a garage but a metal awning, a carport. I knew a lot about architecture, but that was not a word or a structure that I was familiar with. The house had two tall southern pine trees that flanked the entrance and dropped hundreds of small pine cones on the sidewalk and stairs leading up to the front porch. Before I rang the doorbell, a dog inside started barking. Those darn pine cones, I thought. They were everywhere. I couldn't avoid them. They cracked under my shoes as I climbed up the front steps. A few seconds later, the inside door opened, and there stood a comfortably dressed older woman with light-brown skin and gray hair pinned up into a tight bun at the back of her head. She was no more than five feet tall, wore oval wire-rimmed glasses and a green dress under a white apron with evenly spaced small blue flowers. The apron fit snug around her waist.

Smiling as I walked up the stairs, I thought about Grandmother Lulich, who wore a similar apron but never without her black cardigan sweater. I must have been five or six years old the last time I saw my grandmother. In my mind, I heard the melody of an ice cream truck approaching. The driver ringing a set of bells, before slowing down and pulling up to the curb. My grandmother would reach inside the pocket of her apron and pull out a small black coin purse with a metal clasp on the top. Unhooking the clasp, she would pull out a dime and extend her arm in my direction. I'd raise my open hand, palm up, to accept it. She'd gently place the coin in the center of my palm and bend my fingers over the coin to make sure that I didn't drop it. With both of her hands, she'd give my hand a firm squeeze before letting go. She'd do the same for my older brother. Then she'd open the front door and in her Serbo-Croatian English urged us, in a dialect that I barely understood, to hurry and catch the ice cream truck before it left. Her attempts at English sounded like she was angry, accentuating and spitting out the first syllable of every word. Although it sounded harsh, we knew it was her native language colliding with English, because her affection for us was clear.

When Grace Hooks opened the door, I was still smiling as I looked right through her, still lingering in my childhood. Then I looked up and said, "I'm Jody. Barbara sent me."

With the images and sounds of my grandmother fading, I heard Grace Hooks say, "Come in," as she smiled and opened the door.

Unlike my grandmother, Grace Hooks spoke clear English but with the certainty of an East Coast delivery. I had been in Alabama for only two days, but I was surrounded by so many inflections strange to my Midwest upbringing, I wondered if I could grasp all the nuances in the voices and expressions of this new geography.

When I entered through her front door, my eyes widened as I took hold of the elegant furnishings inside. The modest exterior of the house was no match for what I was seeing. Dark wood moldings and solid wood doors framed deep-textured, beige-plastered walls. In front of me, a dark wood Chippendale-style secretary with multiple glass-paned doors on the top and serpentine drawers underneath stood against the wall. To my right, a glass-doored curio cabinet filled with several dozen miniature porcelain shoes. If we had had these things in our house, my father would have sold them. He was not interested in holding on to things that reminded him of the past.

In front of the couch, an oval mahogany coffee table was supported by four dolphins carved out of wood. On the mantel above the fireplace sat an antique gilt spelter clock set in a music box base and covered by a large crystal dome. Orange porcelain jars from Italy. Cobalt blue plates from England. On top of the bookcase was a Wedgwood black basalt water ewer with Triton, the Greek god of the

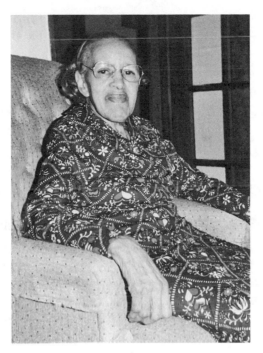

Grace in the den of her home in Tuskegee, 1983.

sea, seated on the shoulder of the spout. Peering in the dining room, I saw, against the wall, a large Jacobean-style great chair covered in deep red upholstery with elegant tassels surrounding the edges. The seat was indented as if Grace sat there often. The chair flanked the window, and elegant thick drapes with a tapestry floral pattern flowed from ceiling to floor. In the center of the dining room was a Sheraton-style mahogany table surrounded by four Regency-style chairs, the upholstery covered in silver-stitched needlepoint in a geometric floral design. These were things that I had only seen in museums. Her house was a museum.

She must have sensed my amazement and said, "These are the things my mother collected. I moved here from Philadelphia to take care of my stepfather after she died in 1958." Then a slight pause. She shifted her body more upright. "My stepfather demanded that dinner be served on my mother's fine Noritake china promptly at 6 each evening except Sundays when we ate at 4." She looked at an empty chair at one end of the table. Her smile disappeared.

She ushered me back into the living room and her smile resumed. Her cheerfulness returned. She took me to a bookcase in the corner and introduced me to her mother's book collection. She handed me a gray book missing its jacket, *The Invisible Man,* by Ralph Ellison. She opened the book and read the inscription. "For the Delaneys, who were most encouraging when encouragement was sorely needed. With many thanks and admiration. Sincerely, Ralph Ellison." She explained that Sadie Delaney was her mother's married name by her second husband. She removed another book from the shelf, *Simple Speaks His Mind.* This one had its jacket cover, although it was worn. "Inscribed especially for Sadie, with all good wishes ever, Sincerely, Langston." She had a 1960 edition of *To Kill a Mockingbird,* the year that it was first published, and many books on art and philosophy. "My mother was a librarian in New York City," she said. "She collected books and antiques."

"This is my mother's house," she emphatically said again as her smile stretched across her face, deepening the creases in her cheeks. She politely excused herself and returned with tea in a silver teapot served on a silver tray. She handed me a cup. When I sat down on the couch, I was careful not to let any spill. Especially since as soon as I sat down, her overweight springer spaniel leaned against my leg. As I lifted the cup to my mouth and drank, the warm tea felt relaxing. It flowed across my tongue and down my throat with ease. My shoulders relaxed, and I slowly let out a comforting sigh. I carelessly reached down and petted her dog. Then I slowly slid the rest of my body into the couch, allowing my back to rest on its cushions. I looked up, smiled, and without saying a word, thought that it would be nice to live here. I would certainly like to get to know Grace Hooks better. She had pride and a sense of family that I was lacking but yearned to be a part of.

That thought didn't last long. I had a few reservations. Grace

Hooks had just told me wonderful and personal things about her mother. What would I say if she asked about mine?

I slowly straightened my back. I slid slightly forward out from the back of the couch until I was at the edge of the seat. When I saw her look my way with raised eyebrows and wide eyes, I knew what was coming.

"Jody," she announced.

I stiffened.

Then she asked, "Where are you from? I'd like to know more about you."

There was so much that I could tell her, and so much that I did not want her to know.

When I was little, my mother loved me so much that she could not let go of me. I hardly left her side. When it was time for me to go to kindergarten, she kept me home with her. When I entered first grade, she cried even though I came home every day for lunch. Some days she would not let me go back to school in the afternoon. When I did go back, she would drink. My mother and father fought. When I was nine, my father had enough. He screamed at her to get out of his life and she did. She committed suicide by drinking antifreeze. On the way to her funeral, we ran over a dog. We did not stop the car to see if the dog was okay. We kept driving to the funeral. Without my mother, my father was incapable of taking care of himself and neglected my brother and me. After high school, I left home and went to college. Sometimes I hurt myself, but it has not happened in a while.

Instead, I simply said Chicago, and nothing more.

At first, the brevity of my response and the pause that followed felt awkward. But it didn't last. Grace liked me, or liked talking to me, or liked telling me the stories of her mother. She was happy to have a passenger while she drove the conversation.

"Here is a letter from Eleanor Roosevelt to my mother. She's thanking her for teaching blind veterans to read and recover." She pressed the letter in my hand to inspect. The signature looked real. Impressive, I thought.

"Here is my mother with Langston. Langston Hughes," she emphasized as if I did not know who Langston Hughes was. She passed the black-and-white photograph over to me.

Langston is standing at the center of a long banquet table. He looks like he is delivering a speech. The audience is laughing, and he has a big smile.

"There's my mother off to his left," Grace said. "She's smiling too. Whatever he said must have been hilarious. Here's my mother in *Look* magazine."

The cover was worn. It had a musty smell of age. A sticky note marked page 29. A cartoon of a librarian with her hair up in a bun was teaching a man with dark glasses to read Braille. Another picture above the cartoon of her captures her mother's face in a graduation cap with a tassel. She wears wire-rimmed glasses.

"She accomplished a lot," she said.

Grace tells me that she has more to show me. At the age of seventy-four, it took some effort for her to get out of her chair, but once up, she moved swiftly, turned around, and with a wave of her hand motioned me to follow. We didn't go far. In the corner of the dining room was an antique Chinese carved side table with an inset pink marble top. On top of it was a burled wood box. It was the size of a large lady's hatbox, about three-quarters of a foot tall and a foot and a half square at its base. A handle came out one side. She grabbed it and gently gave it one crank completely around. She reached over on the other side and pulled on a small brass knob. A flywheel hummed. Gears turned. Tines plunked. And out poured music. Almost comical at first. It had a mechanical quality like a muted calliope. No rubato, no variation in timbre, and no waver in volume. Then she raised the lid, revealing a rotating metal disk as the source of the sound. The melody poured over the brim and filled the room. A sweet harmonious sound. A nostalgic sound. An old lilting tune that pulled out of me a memory of my mother. And I began to talk.

I told Grace that my mother played the piano. That I'd sit next to her on the bench, my legs swinging beneath me because I was fidgety, and I was too small for my feet to reach the floor. She'd press my fingers down over the keys, showing me the scale of C. The following year, she'd teach me how to hold my hands. How to arch my fingers. How to keep my wrists low. How to play the keys with the fleshy part of my fingertips. She'd play along with me and hum the melody to teach me the rhythm. If I became anxious, she'd gently place her hand across the middle of my back, rub small circles just below the yoke of my shirt, and whisper in my ear to relax. In the afternoon with no one else at home but us and the piano, my mother and I made music together in our own world of melodies and laughter.

The music box slowed down. The final notes of Verdi's *La donna è mobile* played and the metal disk stopped. Grace looked at me.

"That was my mother's favorite tune," she said. "Sunday after dinner we would sit and listen to this one and many others."

Grace's face relaxed and her breathing slowed. I imagined that she was revisiting memories of her mother like I was revisiting memories of my mother. She closed the lid and pushed in the stop. The music box would be a gift that Grace would leave me in her will.

The next day at 4:30 p.m., after my classes, Grace Hooks would turn the corner in her 1979 Chrysler and park the car in front of the dormitory where I was staying.

I was sitting on the stoop when she saw me. I waved, stood up, and grabbed a suitcase in each hand. I loaded my suitcases in the back seat, opened the front passenger door, hopped in, and we were off.

I looked at her while she kept her eyes on the road. "How was your day, Mrs. Hooks?" I asked.

"Jody, my friends call me Miss G."

"How was your day, Miss G?" I reiterated.

We both smiled, letting go of formalities. We would become close friends and tell each other our life stories. She would become the family that I always wished for.

24

———

BRAIDING HER HAIR

Coming home to Grace and her beautiful house inspired me to do my best. But there was something wrong. I was happy, but I didn't show it. For the first two months, instead of sharing my day, or making dinner together in the kitchen, or eating dinner with her at the dining room table, I ate yogurt or cottage cheese right out of the refrigerator, right out of the container, or right at my desk. I was getting perfect scores on all my exams, so it was not as if I couldn't have spent some of my time with her. I isolated myself. Maybe out of habit. Maybe out of fear. I can't lose what I never develop affection for. And the pain of loss was still so raw for me. Like my friendships in the past, I was building a wall between them and me before putting in a window.

That all changed the evening Grace asked if I would braid her hair. My bedroom was down the hallway from hers. In the evening, when I heard her call my name, in a soft but imploring voice, I was studying physiology at my desk. I closed my schoolbook and made my way down the hallway.

With each step, the old wood floor creaked and stretched beneath my feet. I remembered the sound because it was quiet that night, no TV, no air conditioner, even her dog, Duke, was asleep. It was odd hearing the movement of my weight across the floor, breaking the night. When I reached her bedroom door, I leaned in, smiled, and answered with a long yes that was more recognizable as a question than a response.

She was sitting in the only chair in the room, a low-back lady's slipper chair with a green cushion. She had taken off her glasses and placed them on top of the dresser. Next to her glasses were a petite pair of silver Victorian fingernail scissors, a matching hand mirror, and a hairbrush.

She looked up at me, hesitated, and then asked, "Would you braid my hair?"

At first, I thought that she was kidding. Why would she ask a twenty-two-year-old man to braid her hair?

Then she looked down at her hands in her lap. Their surface was deeply creased like the rough texture of a crumpled brown paper bag. I never noticed them that way before. The joints connecting the bones of each finger appeared swollen. She gave each hand a gentle caress with the other and then closed her eyes for a few seconds before she let go of her breath.

Seeing her there in pain, I said, "I sure would." Good thing that I went to summer camp the summer after my mother died. It kept my mind occupied, and I learned how to braid strands of nylon into beautiful key chains and other crafts.

I stepped in and sat on the edge of her bed. "Can I slide your chair back toward me?" I said. I pulled her chair in close. As I did, she braced her feet beneath and pushed in my direction. The chair straddled my inner thighs. Her back was now closer to my belly. The back of her head was in front of my chin. I reached forward and removed several hairpins. Her hair slowly swung to the middle of her back. She looked different in the yellow light of the room. With her loose hair and glasses off, she looked softer, contemplative, vulnerable.

She handed me a fancy antique comb. The handle was metal, and the teeth had a muted gray patina.

I gathered her hair from the side of her face and combed it back. I had watched mothers brush their daughters' hair and how their children closed their eyes and contorted their faces. Black children's hair tangled easily. But Miss G's hair was smooth and easy. I was careful and worked slowly. She turned slightly in my direction before saying, "My mother was gentle like you."

"Do you want to know how I came upon all of these beautiful

things, the fine china, the antique furniture, the rare books, the old German music box?" Miss G said.

"You told me. Your mother was an avid collector. When she passed, you inherited the lot."

"No, not the actual things," she gently laughed. "Do you want to know what motivated the collection?"

I gathered up some of her hair and completed a braid. Then rested my right hand lightly on her shoulder and listened.

"The art of collecting was handed down to my mother from her father. In his boyhood, he had been trained to be a gentleman's gentleman in a rich white family in Canada. His mother, my great-grandmother, was also a servant for the same family."

I continued parting her hair. Miss G continued talking.

"Neither of them were born in Canada. She, however, secured her freedom and managed to take him with her through the help of the underground people."

"You mean the underground railroad?"

"Yes, the underground railroad. They always called it the underground people."

I grabbed a portion of her hair and wove another braid.

"At the time my grandfather was barely school age but acquired all the airs and mannerisms of the young fellow to whom he was a valet. As a young adult, he made passage to Rochester, New York. When he arrived, he managed to keep those airs and mannerisms, and he managed to marry my grandmother, who was not of his race but of Indian stock."

"American Indian?" I asked.

"I am not sure. There was like intermingling between Canada and American natives."

She started again. "My grandfather went into the hotel business as a waiter. He moved to Poughkeepsie, where he had the opportunity to become the headwaiter in the largest hotel. He was not only looking for more money, and the new job paid twenty-five dollars per week. He was also hungry for prestige. He found it in Poughkeepsie, New York."

At that time in the early 1900s, Poughkeepsie, New York, knew only the rich. The city folk worked on Wall Street and commuted home from New York City to be with their families.

"My grandfather became the sexton for St. Paul's Episcopal Church. The parish served nothing but the very rich. He was in his element. Sunday morning, he and the rector would greet parishioners. My grandfather, wearing his cutaway coat and winged collar, was at one door; and the rector was at the other door not dressed nearly as nice, I remember my grandfather telling me. My grandfather thought that he was as important as the rector. And to some, he was."

"Grace, I'd love to see a picture of him sometime," I said.

"I'll try and find one," she said. Then she continued. "Parishioners trusted him and relied on him for help and advice. They knew my grandfather admired fine things and thanked him with fine art from their home. In this way, beautiful paintings, floor rugs, and furniture made their way into our house. Our house was the best furnished on the street. I attended his church as a young girl. Being his granddaughter, I too felt that I was someone special. I held my head very high as an aristocrat should."

I had no idea that Grace felt that way. I did not tell her but politely waited for her to finish the story.

"This aristocratic mindset seemingly made my mother want to be better than everyone else. She began collecting when she went to New York City to study to become a librarian. She knew value when she saw it. She would go to flea markets and yard sales and pick up precious art for a fraction of its value. When she came to Tuskegee, Alabama, to work, she brought her collection and many of my grandfather's pieces too. I not only inherited this fine collection, but also the atmosphere that goes with it. I do enjoy the prestige of having it. The collection not only added a cultural atmosphere to my life that suits me well but has carved out a place for me in the community. I am known as Dr. Delaney's daughter with the fine collection."

Sitting on the edge of the bed, I noticed that I was sliding forward. I fidgeted left and then right to secure myself farther on the bed.

"I've tried my best to take care of her things, but from time to time, I've had to sell items due to lack of space and money to give them proper care," Grace said.

Hearing that story, I unfurled the two braids that I had carelessly put together. I picked up the comb and parted her hair into even sections. Using the brush, I ensured that every strand blended perfectly with its neighbors. Holding her hair, I remained silent, remembering my childhood.

After completing the braids, I coiled them flat against her scalp and secured them with a bobby pin. When I completed all the sections, I handed her back the comb and brush. Taking them from me, she put her hand over mine and gave it a gentle squeeze.

I told Grace that I would love to hear more about her family. I had known so little of my family's history that I enjoyed being wrapped up in hers.

She nodded and reminded me, "It is late, and I have taken up so much of your time. I know that you have school in the morning, and I very much appreciate your help."

I walked back to my room, thinking about how much I appreciated living with her.

25

CORNELL

I was up early the next morning. My first class was at 8:00 a.m. Grace's bedroom door was open. On the way out, I peered in. She was asleep, resting on her side. The braids were as I had placed them, coiled and pinned close to her head. I feared that after I went to bed, she would redo them. But I was wrong. I let out a congratulatory sigh of accomplishment.

When I came home after school, her hair was pinned in a bun in its usual fashion, the same as the first day I met her, the same style that she wore every day. The braids were gone, but what lingered was a newfound trust and appreciation for each other and the beginnings of a close friendship.

Instead of eating at my desk and plowing through schoolwork, I sat at the dining room table with Grace. My bowl was filled with cottage cheese—on top was a spoonful of strawberry jam seeping its way between the curds. On the side, a tall glass of cold milk and two slices of bread slathered with peanut butter. I wondered if she would need my help tonight. I hoped that she would.

She smiled when I sat down and then she asked, "How was school?"

"It went well," I said. I am always amazed at how there is so much to know to be a veterinarian. Then I asked her, "How about your day?"

"They want to know if I'm coming to my fiftieth reunion."

"Who wants to know?"

"Cornell University," she said as she pushed the invitation across the table in my direction.

"Cornell University. You graduated from Cornell University! That's amazing. Of course, you should go."

She looked up at me and in silence raised her eyebrows and wrinkled her forehead as if I had said something wrong. Obviously, there was more to this than just the invitation. Then she slid a manila folder to me. Inside was an old newspaper clipping. It was gray and creased as if it were handled often. The *Cornell Daily Sun,* dated December 18, 1929. Folded on the sides and torn across the bottom, emphasizing one article, "Woman's Cosmopolitan Club Conducts Survey on Negro Prejudice in Women's Dormitories."

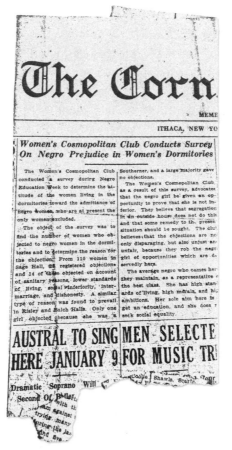

The front page of the Cornell Daily Sun, *Wednesday, December 18, 1929.*

This clipping was from the time she was a student at Cornell. It was yellowed and smudged in areas. From its condition, she must have read it many times.

At first, her voice was shaky. Then she explained why she had reservations. By the end, she was resolute and confident. It became clear as to why she held on to that newspaper article for more than fifty years.

*

"Going through high school as the token Negro had not prepared me for the segregation and isolation I experienced at college," Grace said. "I am not sure if it was my high achievements or my mother's nurturing. I grew up confident, thoroughly ignorant of the forces that would be painful to me later because of the color of my skin."

Grace did most of the talking for a while and I intently listened. "In high school, I was not discriminated against, or at least that was how I felt. I was in the debate club, the dramatic club, and *Le Cercle Français.* I played basketball and other sports. I made top grades. Classmates relied on me for help with their work. Because of my academic standing as a senior, I was encouraged to take the state tuition scholarship exam for Dutchess County, New York. I won second place among all the other high school students, which meant free tuition to Cornell University or any university of my choice in New York.

"Having won the scholarship, you would have thought that I was a celebrity. Reporters came and interviewed me. My picture was in the paper. I was the first and only Black, at that time called Colored, to receive this scholarship. I had a far-off dream of studying medicine and specializing in immunology—something which neither I nor the reporters knew much about. But I knew that I wanted to go to college.

"I first considered Vassar. Vassar was close to home. But Vassar did not admit Negroes. They said that I could attend as long as I was a day student. Vassar wanted me to commute from home on my bike, but I could not live on campus." "Why go to Vassar, if they really didn't want me?" Grace said as if she were asking herself. "Besides, going away to college intrigued me. At the time I had never been further than New York City when I took the Hudson Steamer to visit my mother during her doctorate studies in library science.

"Finally, I decided. I would go to Cornell. My mother's association with rich people for whom she worked ensured that I had all the proper things—a beautiful book bag and notebooks, high nicker shoes, and an inner sense of great accomplishment. They were as excited about properly sending me off as I was about going. But when I arrived on Cornell's campus, as I had at Vassar, the same segregation prevailed. I had no living arrangements. I had expected to live in the dormitory with other students. To my dismay, Cornell did not permit Blacks to live in the dormitory. The Black men worked their way into fraternity houses as waiters and cooks to live near campus. On my first day, I waited for hours to be escorted to the Black community in a little corner of Ithaca. There I stayed in a house with other female Black students. My disappointment could not be covered up. I immediately went to the dean of women to protest this isolation but ran into a brick wall called segregation.

"How dare that squat, big-hipped woman in that floppy black dress tell me where I did and did not belong," Grace Hooks said authoritatively.

I stopped eating my dinner, sat up straight, and listened intently. Then Grace started again.

"I made it quite clear to the dean of women that someone important would hear about this. Someone above her.

"After having said those things, I would have to carry out my threat. I went straight to the president, who informed me that integration had been tried in the past and failed. To make me feel better he said that there was a quota on Jews. I internally murmured, 'and a ban on Blacks.' How was that information supposed to make me feel better? He said that it would probably be lifted someday soon, and he was glad that I made clear my feelings. He was so composed and dignified in his response that he must have been afraid of that squat woman, or my complaint was not the first time he had heard it.

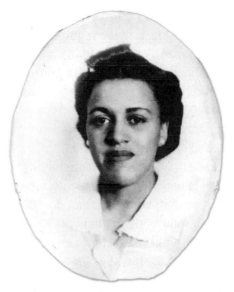

Grace as a student, circa early 1930s.

"By the end of the year, I secured a job in a professor's home near campus. I had gone up and down the streets inquiring if any family needed help. These two older people were sympathetic to my situation. I lived on the same floor as them. My only separation from them and their social life was that I did the cooking. The following year, I got sick, and my appendix burst. I had to leave that job. But when I recovered, I was able to find similar accommodations near campus.

"Even though I was not allowed to live in the dormitory, I was there often. I knew two white girls who were very close. One was poor and worked her way through college. She came from upstate New York from a large family and felt that I was someone who could do no wrong. I do believe that I was her idol. The other girl was Jewish and from a rich family in New York City. She lived in the dormitory and made it her business to invite me constantly to the dining room and her room where we studied. I do believe that she was vindictive and wanted to show me off because her religion and my race were limited to quotas at Cornell.

"Before graduating, I was still keen on living on campus. All undergraduates except Blacks were required to live in the dormitories. I asked the Woman's Cosmopolitan Club for their help. They surveyed the female students in Sage Hall. When the results came out, I was happy and despondent. I was happy because of only twenty-six registered complaints. But those that did complain assumed that I, I mean assumed that female colored students, were unsanitary, socially inferior, and dishonest.

"I was heartbroken," Grace said as she nervously tapped the newspaper article with her finger. "I hope that my teachers did not feel the same. I had just as much right to the same education at Cornell as all the rest of them, but some of them did not see it that way."

"Jody, what do you think? Should I go to my reunion?" asked Miss G.

I sat up with my back against the chair and smiled at her before saying, "I think you've already made your decision."

26

THE LAST LYNCHING

March 1981, at the end of my first year of veterinary school, a nineteen-year-old Black man was found hanging from a tree with a noose around his neck on Herndon Avenue in Mobile, Alabama. He had been beaten and his neck slashed. Adjacent to this infamous tree was the home of Benny Jack Hayes, a high-ranking official of the United Klan of America. The police ignored this juxtaposition and assumed a drug deal had gone wrong, and instead arrested three men hawking illegal drugs, who lived close, but farther down the road.

That evening, when I braided Grace's hair, I asked what she thought of the hanging. "Do you think that those three men killed him and hung his body from a tree?"

She outpoured an abbreviated *hmmm* through tightly closed lips followed by a disapproving shake of her head. The prolonged silence that followed was so thick that I could feel the temperature in the room rise. She was angry but felt sorrow for the things that happened to that man.

Then I realized that this was a modern-day lynching of a Black man, the stuff I read about in history books and thought could never happen in my lifetime. But just did. And like Grace, I felt anger and sorrow at the same time.

For the next few nights, I braided her hair in almost complete silence. When anything was said, Grace did all the talking. The stories she told left me in awe of her profound bravery. But what I couldn't stop thinking about was what a fine job her mother had done in raising her.

*

On the first night, she told me about her trip from New York to Tuskegee on the train.

"The first time I came to Tuskegee was in the summer of 1930, right after graduation from college. My mother secured a Pullman train ticket for me. The train was how people traveled then.

"A Pullman ticket meant that I would have the best accommodations and comforts for the long journey from New York to Alabama. Even though the Great Depression was taking its toll, I had the proper traveling attire and luggage. My hat was small but fashionable and sat on my head with a slight tilt to the left. I carried my white cotton gloves in my hand, because they were too warm to wear, but matched my dress. What made me look older than my age were my grandmother's pearl earrings. They were plain but sophisticated. She handed them to me as I left the house.

"I looked forward to the trip; I had not seen my mother for over a year. Halfway through the journey, after the train departed Washington, D.C.'s Union Station, I was asked, like all the other Blacks, to move to the Jim Crow car in the very front behind the locomotive. It was a habit of mine that when I experienced segregation to suddenly become deaf. I ignored the conductor's request to move. One should not accept such demeaning arrangements without first providing some difficulty," Grace said.

"I was asked to give up my seat again and again. Finally, I acquiesced and got up and made my way, albeit grudgingly, to the Jim Crow car.

"I was not happy. This was not the accommodation my mother paid for. Then one of the steam lines broke in the Jim Crow car. Water was seeping in, and the smoke was annoying. I asked the porter if there was another car available. At first, he ignored me. Then, I stood up in the center of the car and began gathering the attention of the other passengers, all of whom were Black. I encouraged them to band together and complain to our various NAACP organizations.

Our health was being jeopardized, especially those who had little babies, I shouted. When the train stopped at the next station, the porter returned and asked me to follow him. I heard about people who were thrown off the train for protesting. I worried that it was now my turn. But instead, I was escorted out and onto a brand-new Pullman car by myself for the rest of the ride.

"The busboys passing with crackers and drinks were not allowed to sell to me. They must have been told that I had some contagion. When I signaled to them, they refused to stop and veered to the opposite side of the aisle as they approached. Finally, I got up and went back to the Jim Crow car to recruit the others to join me. There was plenty of room, since I was the only passenger, I told them. But they wouldn't budge. They remained obedient to what I thought was an unjust law in a substandard car with a broken steam line while coughing and getting sick.

"Years later, ticket agents were allowed to sell Black folks the tickets for the Pullman cars traveling south of the Mason-Dixon Line, but the railways still managed to maintain segregation. To do this, Blacks were sold tickets with the same series of numbers seating them in designated cars. One time when traveling, there were seven Pullman cars with only Blacks and all the others had only Whites. From then on I ignored my ticket numbers and sat in other cars not designated for Blacks. Since this was after the passage of nonsegregation laws, the conductor had no reason to ask me to move."

When Grace Hooks was done, I asked if she was ever worried for her life.

"The time they took me off the Jim Crow car," she said. "It was very late that night. I thought that they were pulling me off the train. If they left me at the station in the middle of the night a lot could have happened. I feared for my life. I do not think that I would have made it to Tuskegee in one piece."

The next night she told me about her travels on the bus through the South.

"My early travels on the bus were no different," Grace started.

"It was demeaning to know that once the bus crossed that Mason-Dixon Line, I became a second-class citizen.

"On one of my trips to North Carolina, as soon as we crossed over into the South, the driver veered to the side of the road, parked the bus, and demanded that all the Blacks move to the rear. I stood up and made a spectacle of myself. I had written this speech entitled, 'I Am an American.' It was eloquent. I boasted about how my husband and poor brother were off fighting in the war. I didn't have a husband or a brother, but they did not need to know that. So, I just kept going. I told how Blacks had given their blood in the American Revolution so all of you sitting in the front of this bus were free of British rule. And here I am a true American, who would have to give up my seat and move. Beside me, an Italian woman kept asking, 'Do I have to move?'

"I loudly said, 'No. You probably do not have your naturalization papers and you probably are not a true American. But because my skin is black, I am suddenly not good enough to sit with you. I sat here all the way from New York and now I am an undesirable passenger because of the color of my skin.'

"As I gathered up my coat and boots and whatever else I had with me, I kept reciting. Some passengers were quite interested in what I had to say. Some were embarrassed and ducked behind their newspapers. I only wished that I had a recorder with me. My chest puffed out and my shoulders swaggered back and forth. I was proud that I was a Black American, and that I stood up for my race, and against injustice."

I was happy that Grace never had a run-in with the Klan. I am sure that there were some who thought that it would be fitting if she just disappeared. But it must have been quite a sight seeing this petite, five-foot-tall, outspoken Northerner speak her mind, and do it so eloquently.

*

The man hanging from the tree in Mobile, Alabama, was Michael Donald. It took six months for the jury to acquit the three drug dealers of his murder. The jury knew that their indictment was senseless. Besides, there was no evidence, and Donald was a quiet, hardworking individual who never took illegal drugs.

It took two years for the FBI to arrest the real suspects. The event started when a Black man, Josephus Anderson, was tried for shooting a white police officer in Birmingham, Alabama. The trial took place in Mobile, Alabama, where Benny Hayes lived. The jury was unable to reach a verdict. The mistrial exonerated Anderson for shooting a white police officer.

Hayes, a prominent leader of the United Klan of America, interpreted the law how he saw it: "If a Black man can get away with killin' a White man, then a White man should be able to get away with killin' a Black man." Henry Francis Hayes, Benny Hayes's son, and James Llewellyn Knowles took those words to heart. They went out looking for a Black man to kill. Donald just happened to be out that evening walking to the convenience store. He was ambushed. His whereabouts remained unknown until the next morning, when his body was spotted hanging from a tree.

For having resurrected this ancient form of racial terrorism, the courts were not kind to the accused. Knowles was convicted of murder. He was sentenced to life in prison but avoided the death penalty by testifying against Henry Hayes. Hayes was convicted and sentenced to death and was executed on June 6, 1997.

Many years later, the father, Benny Hayes, was indicted for inciting the murder. His court case ended in a mistrial. The jury and judge became sympathetic to his condition when the seventy-one-year-old collapsed in court.

Before this, I never felt unsafe in Alabama. Sometimes when I walked to school, friendly drivers would stop and offer me a ride. After the death of Michael Donald, I was more cautious about getting into someone's car unless I was familiar with the driver.

One car trip, however, put me on high alert. My classmate's mother unexpectedly died, and he needed a ride to the Atlanta airport, a hundred-mile road trip from Tuskegee. I borrowed Grace's car. Vicki, my lab partner, came with me. We drove to Atlanta with plenty of time for our classmate to catch his flight. We were in such a rush to get back, because we had a major exam the next morning, that I didn't notice the gas gauge was sitting near empty. As we approached Opelika, thirty miles from home, the car sputtered. Before it stopped, I was able to park it on the shoulder of the road, yards from an exit ramp. It was dark, almost 10:00 p.m., and the interstate had no street-lights. We got out and walked up the exit ramp hoping to find a gas station. Instead, we came up into a poorly lit residential area with a few homes and many open fields. We looked at each other and won-dered if we should go back to the car and hope that the state patrol would rescue us or knock on the door of one of those houses and ask for help. The fear of missing an exam pushed us into a potentially compromising position. We knocked on the door of the house clos-est to the exit ramp. The porch light came on and the door slowly opened. An older white man stood on the other side of the door. I could not see past him because there were no other lights on in the house. After explaining our predicament, I asked if we could use his phone to call a friend for help. This was the 1980s, and cell phones were not available. The homeowner, in a deep Southern dialect, said that we should be more careful and warned us about the dangers of being out late after sunset. Then he pointed to the phone on a table near the door. We had to step inside, which made me nervous, but we needed to call for help. We quickly called Carlos, our lab partner, thanked the man for letting us use his phone, and walked back to the car. Remembering the man's warning, we got in the car and locked the doors. Only after Carlos arrived did our anxiety go away. Carlos put gas in the car, and we made it back safely.

I could not sleep that night. I was rattled by what could have hap-pened and needed the extra time to study. I thought a lot about Carlos. We were good friends. I was pleased that under all the stress of being stranded that I was able to remember his phone number. How could I forget; we talked all the time.

27

THE GIFT

Completing the first year of my veterinary education had many surprises. I was at the top of my class academically. I received an A in every course, which meant that I received free tuition during the coming year. I received a lot of encouragement from classmates, instructors and staff, and of course from Grace Hooks. I enjoyed the newly acquired confidence that I did not have when I arrived.

I stayed in Tuskegee the following summer. I needed to fulfill a requirement in animal nutrition that I couldn't take during the normal school year. Thinking back, I don't remember anything that I learned that summer. But I do remember how unbearably hot it was. Every day the temperature rose above one hundred degrees. The class was primarily outside doing fieldwork. We visited cow and goat farms. I would come home and fall over the bed exhausted and not get up and eat until sunset when the heat dissipated. I managed a short break before the beginning of the next semester and went to Chicago.

Being home made me realize just how much I missed Grace Hooks. I called her often and anticipated my return.

When I did make it back, she was at the front door to greet me, with open arms and a huge smile. I looked up at her and noticed immediately that she had cut her hair.

It looked smart, combed back behind her ears with a curl at the neckline. I held on to my smile. I reached forward and hugged her and told her it looked nice. I am sure that she sensed my disappointment no matter how hard I tried to hide it.

Combing and braiding her hair was how we spent our evenings. Through her, I learned about the world. I learned about Grace and how much I appreciated her.

Taking care of her at night was how I began to love myself. It was just the two of us and I wasn't feeling lonely anymore. I was not competing with anybody or trying to please anybody. I was learning to trust again. This simple task made a huge difference in how I saw the rest of the world.

I should have known that the length of her hair would have little to do with our friendship. And it didn't. But she could have told me before cutting it. There were still times that she needed my help in the evening. From then on, our chats were heart-to-heart, face-to-face, and eye-to-eye.

I was indebted to Grace. She welcomed me into her home as if I had always belonged there. She shared her lessons for living a life without regret. She demonstrated that purpose and hard work lead to happiness. She loved me as a parent loved a son. She filled so many holes in my life that were empty that I had to do something special for her. As the Christmas holiday approached, I began thinking about a gift I could give her. I wanted to give her something special.

On the weekend before my finals, I asked Miss G if I could borrow her car. After she handed me the keys, I drove to Montgomery, the closest big city. In the Eastdale Mall, I found a small store that sold art glass and exotic pieces of wood crafted into bowls, penholders, and other common items. At first, I didn't see anything that suited me. As I walked farther back into the store, my eyes zeroed in on a beautiful wood box with a hinged top. It was the perfect size for holding letters, ten inches long and six inches wide. The sides were stained a dark forest green that accentuated the grain of the wood. Teardrops, leaves, and circles were carved into the top and stained deep red, orange, and black. It was just what I had imagined. I told the clerk that I would buy it and asked if the store sold calligraphy pens.

After final exams and at dinner the night before my return to

Chicago for the Christmas holiday, I presented the gift to Grace. She carefully removed the white ribbon and bow, and then the red wrapping paper with reindeers wearing Christmas wreaths.

She slid out the box and said, "Oh, this is beautiful."

"Open it," I said.

She opened the box. In the bottom was a folded sheet of medium-weight beige paper. She lifted the paper and unfolded it.

"It is a poem I wrote for you," I said. Grace had so many beautiful things that I knew that anything that I could buy would be senseless.

Grace began silently reading the poem.

"Can I read it to you?" I asked.

She smiled, nodded, and handed me the poem.

> *I held her hair between my fingers*
> *Imagined it once dark and full*
> *Now long and silver, and full of stories*
>
> *Never before had I touched her hair*
> *Always pulled back, lifted, bunned and pinned*
> *Never before had I seen it relaxed and loose*
> *She trusted onto me the duty that her aging hands*
> *   could no longer hold.*
>
> *I spread my fingers and pulled my hands to the very tips*
> *   of her hair,*
> *Feeling the surfaces of every road she traveled,*
> *Every challenge that shaped her,*
> *And every love that she once vowed to kept silent.*
>
> *I held her hair between my fingers*
> *Separating sections of silk to braid*
> *Sections below, lifted and crossed, and blended and joined*
> *Strengthening each strand with the company of others*

Never before had I experienced such closeness
I reached out and gently held her hair in the palm of my hands
Closed my eyes and imagined it once dark and full
Now long and silver, and full of stories.

We sat there looking at each other. Her eyes welled up. Seeing her so touched by my words, I teared up too.

She reached over and I handed her the poem. She laid it on the table and lightly rubbed her hand over its surface while looking up at me. Then she picked it up, looked at it again, and pressed it lightly over her heart.

She told me that she had never been honored so gracefully before. I told her that I had never met someone so deserving before.

Every Christmas that followed, and sometimes on her birthday, I made sure to add to the collection. To my surprise, she responded with poetry and essays of her own. Some were new and some were pieces that she had written earlier. All of them, whether from me or her, were deeply moving, immensely appreciated, and genuinely heartfelt.

28

THE LETTER

On a warm Saturday afternoon in April, I decided to sit outside on the front porch and catch up on my studies. That day, the winds carried a cooler than expected breeze for an Alabama spring. I opened my physiology book and read the chapter on the respiratory system, an assignment that I had promised myself to complete the week before. I sat there for less than a half hour before the sun vanished behind an overcast sky of gray clouds. Off in the distance, the rumbling thunder was edging its way in my direction. When lightning crisscrossed the sky above me, I knew that it was time to head inside for safety. On the way in, I passed Grace, sitting on the couch and going through the day's mail. She barely looked up as I passed.

I had not called home for several months and decided to check in. My father picked up the phone. After I said hello and before I could ask how he was doing, he told me that my brother was angry with me.

I had not seen my brother for at least two years. I made a conscious effort to avoid him.

Then my father said, "Gary found a letter in your bedroom."

What type of letter, I asked.

"It was sealed and addressed to him," my father said.

Then I remembered. I wrote that letter when I was leaving for college. I was angry with my brother for taking my bike and wrecking it. Instead of apologizing, he said that it was not my bike anyway because Dad paid for it.

"Jody, you wrote that when I die, Gary might as well jump in the grave with me because you were not going to take care of him," said my father.

I was becoming irritated. What was Gary doing in my bedroom? Besides, Gary could learn to take care of himself if given the opportunity.

I told my father that I wrote that letter to myself and that I never intended to send it.

Of course, at the time that I wrote it, I meant every word. The way my brother beat the crap out of me when we were growing up, I didn't owe him anything, especially not my kindness. Then I thought, why am I being accused of upsetting my brother when I did everything possible to just stay out of his way. I became angry. I blurted into the phone. "What did you expect me to write? Gary hangs the dog because it will not follow his commands. He throws me out of the house in the winter without my coat. He hits me so hard in the chest that I fall over backward and hit my head. You had to take me to the emergency room. Remember." My voice was now shaky and high-pitched.

The thunder roared and the lightning cracked. Then I screamed into the phone. "You never said anything to him. I felt as if you did not care how cruel he was. To the dogs. Or to me. I felt like you did not care about me. I felt like you did not love me." My voice stumbled over those last words. The phone was silent for what felt like an eternity. Then I heard a click on the other end.

Grace got up from the couch in the living room. In between each step was a knock on the wood floor from her cane as she approached. Before she reached my bedroom, she said, "Jody, are you okay?"

Boom. A loud crash of thunder shook the house seconds after sparks of lightning lit up the interior spaces. The windows rattled as rain pelted the glass. Then the electricity went out, throwing us into darkness.

Grace stopped where she was. I looked into the hallway and recognized her silhouette and how the shadows concealed the features of her face. I hoped the shadows did the same for mine. I didn't want her to see how angry I had become.

"I am okay, Miss G. Are you okay?" I said.

Boom. The thunder shook the house again.

"Really, I am okay," I said louder and in her direction. But I was not okay. In my father's eyes, I could not do anything right. I was not angry with my father. I loved my father. It was my brother I despised.

"I am okay too," said Grace. "When the electricity went out, I detoured into my bedroom. I'm going to lie down until this storm blows over. These old bones need a rest."

When the electricity came back on, we had dinner together. It was as if we were unshaken by the day's events. While eating, we talked about the weather, if the rain affected her arthritis, and what we really thought about President Reagan. I avoided bringing up the conversation that I had had earlier with my father. I was too embarrassed to mention that I got all worked up over a letter that I wrote six years ago.

29

THE IRONY OF IT ALL

For years, I had questioned how such a small amount of antifreeze could kill my mother. I knew my mother's emotional state when she drank it. And I witnessed her vomiting and the pain that followed. But I needed to know more. I needed to know why she suffered so intensely. I needed to know at the most basic and scientific level what went awry in her body. Was there anything that could have saved her, or helped her, or helped me?

Although I had been questioning, I was not ready to know until years after her death.

While studying physiology, I submerged myself in the information. I wanted to know what her body went through the night she drank antifreeze. However, it was not until my toxicology class a year later that I understood the irony of it all. Nevertheless, I now knew. By drinking antifreeze, her kidneys completely shut down. Because the toxins could no longer leave her body, she suffered, and without slipping from sobriety, she would seal her fate.

The toxic ingredient in antifreeze is ethylene glycol, a colorless, odorless, sweet-tasting chemical. It is small, one-third the size of glucose. It is made of two carbon atoms, six hydrogen atoms, and two oxygen atoms. Ethylene glycol is innocuous as long as it is not broken down into smaller compounds by the liver. If my mother did not have a liver, which is impossible to live without, the poison would have had no effect. It would have been rapidly absorbed through the stomach, passed through the kidneys, and exited in her urine. We would have not noticed its presence if it were not for the giddy tipsiness it causes and the increased urine volume it creates on its way out. But an enzyme in my mother's liver would change ethylene glycol's shape and its safe exit, and instead transform it into something deadly.

The liver receives blood from two sources. One is oxygen-rich and comes from the heart and the lungs and supplies vital nutrients and energy for the liver to thrive and function. The other blood supply is oxygen-poor and comes from the digestive tract. This blood supply carries digestive nutrients that need to be converted into usable compounds, and digestive waste products that must be disarmed. In other words, all the blood from the stomach and intestine goes through the liver first for processing before entering the general circulation.

The liver accomplishes this feat by housing enzymes to break down nutrients and waste products. One family of enzymes, the alcohol dehydrogenases, were well acquainted with my mother. They understood her intentions, her mistakes, her weaknesses, and her recidivism. They understood her drinking problem. They knew how to break down ethanol in the booze she drank, into small compounds that are utilized as food.

Alcohol dehydrogenase adapted to my mother's lifestyle. It knows that its survival depends on my mother's survival. It wants to protect her. So it stays vigilant and stands guard. It waits for her depression and loneliness, her triggers for drinking. And when she does, it gets excited. It undulates and lures the ethanol within reach. And just when the ethanol is about to start its party on my mother's nervous system, alcohol dehydrogenase locks onto its form, draws it in close, tightly fastens its arms around it, and begins a party of its own. It rips the hydrogen atoms off before passing the injured ethanol to a series of coconspirators who continue the deconstruction and division until all that remains are harmless molecules of water and carbon dioxide. My mother has to drink more and quicker to numb the depression and loneliness that shelter inside. And so she does. She drinks and drinks until the liver is beat. Its defenses spent. And the intruder wins.

But when my mother filled her drinking glass with antifreeze and drank it, the outcome was different. It was as if my mother had sent a

Trojan horse to each alcohol dehydrogenase enzyme. The difference between ethylene glycol and ethanol is minimal, a single atom of oxygen. As the ethylene glycol seeped through the wall of her stomach and into her bloodstream, alcohol dehydrogenase would not recognize the difference. It would begin to vibrate and lure the unsuspecting imposter into the same dance that it so joyously enacted with ethanol. But instead of creating harmless end products, it would be a dance of death. Alcohol dehydrogenase would rip ethylene glycol of its hydrogen arms and then pass the injured molecule to its coconspirators where they eagerly completed the deconstruction. Instead of ending up with harmless molecules of water and carbon dioxide, the process will unveil villainous aldehydes, acids, and oxalates. The kidneys would struggle to rid the body of these annihilators. They would not be outsmarted. Aldehydes are a strong irritant causing cell death. Acids shift the neutrality of the blood. Actively charged oxalates rapidly latch onto minerals in the blood, forming crystals, shutting down my mother's kidneys and turning them into stone.

*

I assumed that my understanding of her suicide was complete. I thought that my attachment to the pieces and the process was loosening its effect on me. But I was wrong.

In toxicology class, the instructor lectured on antifreeze poisoning. I held the pencil in my hand and wrote down everything he said. But I already knew the toxic principles. I knew the chemical structures. I knew the normal physiology and how ethylene glycol disrupted it. And I knew firsthand the consequences if the process could not be stopped.

I slowly lifted my head and listened. Or hardly listened. I did not want to hear it again. My mind drifted back in time. But as soon as I heard the instructor say, "The sweet taste of antifreeze makes it a common poison used to commit suicide," I sat up straight and stared into the instructor's face. He looked back at me. I feared that he knew. I had not said a word to anyone about it. How would he know that my mother committed suicide by drinking antifreeze? How did anyone know? That was my story, and I kept it to myself.

And then I heard, "To block the toxic effects of ethylene glycol, administer grain alcohol."

The pencil in my hand loudly cracked in two as I tightly closed my fist.

"The affinity of alcohol dehydrogenase is one hundred times greater for ethanol than ethylene glycol. If you saturate the enzyme with booze, ethylene glycol would remain intact and harmless and get excreted in the urine," said the instructor.

The irony of it all. My shoulders slumped. The night my mother drank antifreeze, everything was out of place and out of order. The inevitability of her death was juxtaposed so close to the possibility of her survival. The close relationship of the pieces, bad and good at the same time, was overlooked. Yet the timing was all wrong. All my mother had to do was to be her drunken self. The one thing that I detested and tried to get her to stop. All she had to do was feel the loneliness and pain that sent her to those places, those dark places. Those places in which the only way out was drinking.

She was more familiar with the antidote than any of us. All she had to do was reach for a drink. It was her way of life. Yet, this one time, this final time, she was faithful enough, or shameful enough, or sane enough, or strong enough, or hurt enough to say no. If only she had been weak enough to say yes. If only we had been less critical and more accepting of her drinking, maybe she could have saved herself. We all needed help. We all could have handled that better.

30

———

THE NEIGHBORHOOD VET

Thelma called me in Alabama to tell me that she had arranged a summer job for me. During the past seven years when I had been away at college and vet school, Thelma had become quite the animal whisperer. She fed the stray cats in the neighborhood. Whenever they spotted her in the yard, they came running and rubbed up against her legs. Thelma returned the affection by dispersing treats in large quantities. When a stray dog crossed her path, she decided to bring that one home, making it a member of the family. Before doing so, she took the dog to the neighborhood vet clinic for a checkup and shots. During the appointment, Thelma mentioned that her son was in veterinary school. I'm not sure what she said after that, but the next thing I knew was that I had a summer job assisting the veterinarian in our neighborhood clinic.

I accepted the opportunity. I saw the clients before the veterinarian checked in. He allowed me to assist in multiple surgeries, many I did by myself with only his supervision. However, there was one appointment that I was not prepared for. I decided to spay the family dog, a deep-chested, seventy-pound Doberman. She was anesthetized, on the surgical table, and draped when I made the first incision. I was too timid. I made a hundred little cuts when I should have made a deep longer incision. With my hands submerged in her abdominal cavity, I could not find the reproductive tract. I hunted and hunted. Her other organs slipped between my fingers, but each time I came up empty-handed. I could not find the uterus. Where could it be, I thought.

To locate the uterus, veterinarians use a spay hook. The utensil reminded me of a prop I had seen in old vaudeville movies. When the act failed and the crowd booed, out came a large hook that corralled the entertainer around the neck and whisked him off the stage. A similar hook, only much smaller, is used to corral the uterus. With my hands gloved and buried deep inside our dog's abdomen, I went fishing. I inserted the hook, glided it along the inside wall, twisted it so that the opening faced the midline of our family pet, and lifted it. The hook came up empty. I tried again. Still empty. Then I entered on the other side. The intestines sloshed and fell against my hand. When the hook came up, it was still empty. I did not give up. I tried again and again. I asked for a stool to stand taller and look inside. All I saw were dark red organs billowing up. Not one of them was the uterus. The room was getting warm, and I felt dizzy. Finally, I asked for help. The female veterinarian stepped in to finish the job, but not before admonishing me. "You do not do surgery on your own pet," she said. I agreed. I felt awful. I also worried too much about making a mistake, about making the incision too large, about creating unnecessary pain and discomfort. I stepped away from the surgery and watched from a distance. She quickly found the uterus and ovaries, removed them, and closed the abdomen. Our dog recovered and did well despite my inexperience and poor judgment.

As I worked in the clinic, my surgical skills and my confidence continued to improve so much that Thelma convinced me to neuter all the stray cats that she had been feeding all summer. I was frightened, but we made a plan. Thelma collected supplies from work. I didn't ask how she got them, but over several weeks, she brought home disposable laceration packs, surgical scrubs, sterile gloves, and suture. I mentioned to her that the veterinarian injected antibiotics at the end of each surgery. The next week she brought home an opened bottle of ampicillin. I stored it in the refrigerator to keep it fresh. When I mentioned that the plastic utensils in the disposable laceration pack did not close properly, she brought home metal needle holders, a good pair of surgical scissors, shiny tissue forceps that looked like tweezers, and more packages of suture, this time with the needles already attached. That was when I knew that we were really doing this.

When I went to work the following Monday, the clinic had a full schedule of appointments, including four surgeries, two castrations and two spays, all of them cats. I prepared for the surgeries in the morning, setting out the surgery packs and drawing up all the injections. At noon, we closed the hospital for several hours to complete the operations without interruptions. When one of the cats didn't show up, I explained that my mother wanted me to neuter the strays that lived in the alley. I told the veterinarian that I had all the supplies except the anesthesia. Since one cat was a no-show for its surgery, I asked if I could use the injectable drugs to anesthetize the stray cats. At first, he hesitated. But he felt that I could be trusted. For two weeks when he was preparing for a wedding, I was in charge of running the entire clinic, including the relief veterinarian, whose medical skills I did not trust. I had to step in and modify patient care that I surmised he botched. In the end, the veterinarian who hired me said yes and then reminded me that I needed to keep a record of all anesthetic drugs used. "It is the law," he said.

Neutering the male cats was easy. Thelma held them. I injected the valium-ketamine-acepromazine cocktail into the muscles along the back. If the cats were calm, I injected smaller amounts into a tiny vein in the front leg. Within minutes, the first cat was out and breathing quietly on its own. I shaved the hair over the testicles. I cleaned the skin with the pink surgical soap and then wiped the skin with iodine-soaked gauze. Thelma held the cat, keeping the tail and legs out of the way. I donned a pair of sterile gloves and held the scalpel firmly in one hand. Using my other hand, I grabbed the scrotum and pushed one testicle toward the surface. I made a half-inch incision through the skin. Not a drop of blood percolated up. I made the incision deeper. White flesh bulged from underneath the opening. I squeezed harder. The testicle popped through the opening like edamame popping out from its pod. The testicle was still attached by vessels at one pole and a ligament at the other. I clipped the ligament. With the ligament in one hand and the testicle with its attached vessels in the other hand, I make a knot with the two as if

I were tying my shoe. The knot descended into the incision, ending the blood supply to the testicle. I tied a second knot and then used my scalpel to free the testicle. I did the same procedure on the other side, and the cat woke up a eunuch.

I was nervous doing surgery without supervision. Thelma is a great nurse, but she had no surgical skills. I cradled the cat in my lap until I saw him moving on his own. I lightly touched his nose, and he stuck his tongue out and licked the spot that I just tapped. I handed him over to Thelma and instructed her to rub his fur with a warm towel. In response, the cat stretched his body. He was recovering. I felt relieved.

For my next surgery, I spayed a female orange tabby. I stroked the cat's head and told her what we were about to do and that she was in great hands. She looked up at me as if she understood. I injected the anesthetic, and she quickly relaxed into a deep sleep. I was especially careful with her. She was very petite. I laid her on her back and secured her forelimbs in front of her head and her hind limbs behind her butt. This exposed her belly. I shaved the belly and disinfected the skin. To get into the abdomen, I knew that I had to make a deep incision. The scalpel slid easily as it cut through the skin. Below was the linea alba, which literally means white line. It is a fibrous tissue that provides strength to the abdominal wall. Using the scalpel, I stabbed the linea and made a small hole. I inserted one blade of the scissors through the hole and cut in a straight line in the direction of the navel opening into the abdomen. I could see the intestines and urinary bladder. I thought back on our Doberman's surgery and how I was not fully prepared. I swallowed hard and reminded myself of the anatomy. The uterus would be beneath the intestine. Stay calm, I whispered. It will be okay. I used the spay hook and on the first approach fished up the uterus. I examined it to make sure that I had the correct structure. I traced the organ up to the ovaries. I tied off above the ovaries on one side and then the other, not just with one knot but with several. Then I tied off below the base of the uterus. I carefully cut free the reproductive tract and lifted it out of the abdomen.

I closed the abdomen in two layers, an interior row of sutures zipping up the linea alba and another below the skin. This time I used absorbable sutures on the underside so that Thelma would not have to capture the cat again to remove skin sutures. These ligatures would seal and dissolve over time. I gave the cat an antibiotic shot and let her recover in a box of warm towels from the dryer. I sat over her, petting her head and gently massaging her closed eyelids. Then she blinked, a sign that she was recovering from the anesthesia. I exhaled in relief.

"It would be better to keep the cats indoors overnight," I told Thelma. I wanted to make sure that they had a good night's sleep in a clean area and without too much activity. I wanted them to eat a hefty breakfast in the morning before being released. That night, I sat with all the cats while they recovered and offered them small licks of food from my finger. I worried that they would be frightened now that they were confined to a small kennel instead of being free in the yard.

The next morning all the cats were active and playful. I hoped that neutering them would prevent their fighting or, better yet, that a neighbor would take one in and care for it as a new family member.

I released the cats one at a time. Each one darted through the yard and disappeared into the bushes except one. The orange tabby stayed nearby, turned around, and brushed up against my leg. I reached down and petted her. She welcomed the affection by stretching up into my hand.

By the time I returned to school at the end of August, I had logged in 103 surgeries, 96 with the supervision of a veterinarian, and 7 on the kitchen table with Thelma assisting. All were a success.

31

CHRISTMAS 1983

Beginning my fourth year of veterinary school, I prepared my intern-ship application. An internship is often a stepping stone to specialty training and an advanced degree. I considered a career in pathology. I studied architecture in high school and college and acquired an appreciation of anatomic structure and its relationship to function. Although an internship was not a prerequisite for advanced training in pathology, it was important to have a deep understanding of the clinical disease when the specimen is alive before seeing it under a microscope lens or on a postmortem table.

The application process was the harbinger of something more serious, the completion of my veterinary education. I would soon be a doctor, and moving away from someone I deeply cared for, Grace Hooks.

That year I didn't go back to Chicago at Christmas: I spent it with Grace. With my last exams of the fall semester completed, I helped clean the house. We still had several days before Christmas. Together we planned a traditional feast, turkey with stuffing, cranberry sauce, and green beans. We made a list for our trip to the grocery store. I mentioned that we should buy the pumpkin pie, so we did not have to make that too. She agreed.

On the way out of the house to get groceries, she handed me the car keys. It was her car; we were merely switching the seating arrange-ment. I was behind the wheel and she was enjoying the view. I looked over and asked if she had her seat belt on. She pulled it up from the side and handed it to me and I buckled her in. When we got to the store, I released the latch of her seat belt and carefully let it fall to her right, exited the driver's side of the car, and opened the passenger door for her. I helped her up and handed her walking cane to her. I motioned the crook of my right arm in her direction, and with her left hand, she embraced my arm. Together, we proudly walked into the store.

She pushed the grocery cart and I collected the goodies. As I was finding lettuce, cucumbers, and tomatoes in the produce section, Grace met up with a familiar face.

"Grace, I never knew you had a son!" the woman said. She looked a few years younger than Grace.

Grace said, "Yes, and it is so good to have him home at Christmas."

After I placed the produce in the cart, I nudged her and we both laughed. I didn't ask Grace why she didn't set her friend straight. I already knew why. Grace had become as close to a mother as I would ever find, and she needed a son.

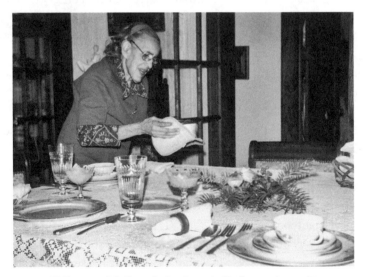

Christmas with Grace in her home in Tuskegee, circa 1983.

32

OUR MOTHERS

I would eventually tell Grace of my mother's death. And although she knew my mother was dead, I told her very little of the details, only that I was nine when it happened. Near the end of my veterinary education, I would hear much about her mother's death, in great detail.

"My mother's death was sudden" was how Grace started one evening. I could tell by the look on her face that she was reliving a painful part of her past. So I was careful not to interrupt.

"It was a heart attack," said Grace. She paused and then continued. "I was living in Philadelphia. I was called by the telegraph company that a message had come through the phone, but the connection was not working properly, and the message was delayed for more than four hours. By then, one of my mother's best friends had phoned the news in a very proper and serene voice.

"At the time I lived alone," said Grace. "There was no one with me to whom I could express my shock and my sorrow and my regret for not having talked to her recently or for not being there when she died. I gathered what I needed for a short trip and took the next plane to Tuskegee.

"When I arrived, there was a great deal of bustling about. The plans were already underway for all the things that needed to be done when one dies, especially if one was prominent. I remembered that my mother had left a letter stating just how she wanted to be funeralized. I found it among her effects. She wanted to be 'in state' at the Veterans Administration Hospital for one day. She wanted certain verses to be read from the Bible and her favorite hymn to be sung.

She was dressed in the special attire that she requested. I made her hair in the manner in which she always wore it.

"My stepfather had just about collapsed and could do nothing but sit with his face in his hands. There were so many people about the next day that I had to get away for a few moments of quiet. An old friend, a doctor, took me to his office, where I had a few moments of quiet. I was able to gather my composure and keep it through the services, until the end. Then I cried and cried and cried.

"The house was so empty after the funeral even with my stepfather there. My mother was so vivacious. Her electrifying presence was sorely missed. Even today I feel her presence, and I am not ashamed to say that I find myself mimicking some of her mannerisms.

"My stepfather lived on eight years after my mother's death. He managed to be a part of and separate from the world about him. He had an uncanny way of doing everything the same as he had done in the twenty-five years of their married life. Until he became ill, everything was done by him nearly at the same time and in the same way. For a time, I tried to keep the pattern of my mother's life with him by setting the table just the same, having dinner at the same hour, keeping up the furniture and all of the little things that counted in his surroundings. But it did not seem to add much to his happiness. I found him going to the cemetery quite frequently, standing and talking to my mother's grave.

"I had a big birthday party for him and invited many of his friends, neighbors, and my mother's friends. He did not enjoy it, although I went through a great expense to make it an attractive and lively party. He objected to me using the very fine glass and delicate finger bowls. I just went on using these things, thinking that it would make him comfortable if he saw them being used. After a while, my stepfather's mind began to show signs of weakness, and he began to find great fault in me although I was steadily trying to please him."

I didn't interrupt Grace, but at that moment, I looked away briefly and realized that we had more in common, our search for parental love and approval. I also realized that it may never happen or there may come a time when my father would be unable or not be here to provide it.

Grace continued, "My relief from this type of pressure was to be active in community work. Having been certified as a social worker, I had a full life and felt satisfied by helping others. But I wanted to share my discoveries and accomplishments with him. He would not hear of it. I did little things to make him happy. I'd bake gingerbread on Fridays and serve it with applesauce as my mother had done before. I provided him with a comfortable reclining chair. He complained that it was not long enough for him to stretch out and went to bending over his bed to do his crossword puzzles. He was an avid philatelist and occupied most of his day with stamps and crossword puzzles. It was uncanny how he kept himself aloof in work of his own. I knew that he was trying to continue life with mother, although she had passed.

"When my stepfather passed in 1966, it was necessary for me to construct a new life for myself in this house, which was completely furnished with my mother's treasures, and too large to live in alone. Friends and neighbors were very kind in trying to keep me company, but they soon realized that I was going to survive somehow on my own.

"There was a young lady who confided in me. She was having difficulty with her parents. She and her boyfriend would sit out on campus and talk. She would get home late for dinner or stay out later than her folks thought that she should. This created constant friction between her and her parents. I knew her parents quite well and asked if their daughter might live with me. She would be my foster child, and I, her older companion. Not in a legal sense, but in a mutual trust between me and her, and her parents. She had a room of her own and paid a little for her conveniences.

"Since that time, many have occupied that back bedroom. Most of them students of Tuskegee University. Some have gone on to be doctors and administrators. One is a high-ranking official in the army. Two have worked at the veterinary school. Most developed close friendships with me and I adopted them, but some were just renters. Jody, and then you came along. It's been almost four years. It's been a joy having you here. You helped me during my second hip replacement. And you were so kind to Duke. I am not sure that I will be able to get along without you. I am going to miss you terribly."

I reached across the dining room table and lightly placed my hand over hers. We were silent, a profound silence in anticipation of the immense distance that would soon separate us.

33

GRADUATION

Graduation at Tuskegee University was always on Mother's Day. Sunday, May 13, 1984, would be no different. After four years of veterinary school, I graduated first in my class. Grace Hooks was in the audience to cheer me on as I marched in the procession, shook the hand of the university's president, and received my diploma with the highest honors. My father and Thelma didn't attend. The distance between Chicago and Tuskegee was 793 miles, five hours by plane, twelve hours by car, and eighteen years in the making after my mother died. But his absence was not unexpected. He had not attended my high school graduation and showed no interest in seeing me graduate from college, both of which were geographically closer.

After graduation, Grace too would be gone, but only for a short departure. She was having hip replacement surgery the next day and needed to check into the hospital the night before the operation.

After all the pomp and circumstance, I came home to an empty house except for Grace's dog, Duke, who greeted me with enthusiasm and slobbery kisses as I opened the door. He was happy to see me, although possibly happier to have his dinner. I was happy to see him too. The house was quiet. We kept each other company for a week until Grace returned from the hospital.

I delayed my trip home to Chicago to assist Grace in her recovery, but we both knew that soon I would have to leave. I accepted an internship at the University of Minnesota and was expected to arrive by the end of June. As my departure date approached, it would be difficult for Grace and me to say goodbye, but we tried not to think about it. Instead, we spent our time reminiscing and enjoying each other's company.

Remember the night we went searching for Duke. You woke me up after midnight. You were so worried. He escaped from the backyard and wandered off. You handed me a flashlight and we got in the car, you in your nightgown and me in shorts and a T-shirt. You drove up and down Bibb Street. We lowered the windows and hollered his name over and over. I scanned the side streets and the neighbors' yards with the flashlight. Duke was all black except for a few white patches on his face. I didn't think we were going to find him. It was difficult to see anything in the middle of the night. I was amazed that your neighbors didn't call the police on us. When I spotted him and called his name, he came running to the car, and when I opened the door, he jumped in the back seat. Duke was obedient when he wanted to be. I couldn't fall asleep that night after all the excitement. I am sure that you must have had the same problem.

"Of course I remember," Grace said. "That was kind of you to help me. I was frightened of losing him."

It was a joy grocery shopping with you every weekend. You taught me much about community. Each trip, you picked up something for someone else less fortunate than us. They were surprised when we arrived at their door bearing gifts.

"I had to take care of Barbara's sister," Grace said, "she had sickle cell anemia. I knew her when she was a little girl." "And Gertrude, she was one of my closest friends. When she started losing her memory, I wanted to help in any way that I could."

You also showed me how to cleverly skirt around the truth. Your friends would say, Grace, I didn't know that you had a son. Instead of telling the truth, you'd say how wonderful it was to have me home.

"It was none of their business anyway," Grace said smiling. Besides, "I didn't lie."

I smiled too. She was right. She was not lying, but she was not exactly telling the truth either.

I got up out of the chair and sat on the floor next to her. I reached over and through her socks gently massaged the foot on the side of her new hip. Duke came over and helped by leaning into both of us.

Grace closed her eyes and murmured, "Thank you."

"Can I play the music box?" I asked.

"Of course," said Grace.

I slowly opened the lid. "Sweet By and By" was set to play. I wanted something less Christian and more soothing. I replaced it with the song "Long, Long Ago." Unexpectedly, the slower pace and lower tones filled the room with melancholy. I hovered over the music box, looking down at the disk turning. Its patina was mottled and tarnished: signs of old age and having been selected many times before. The song played through a few verses, and as it slowed down, the lilting pace of the melody tugged on memories of our time together, and then stopped without completing the song. I wound the crank several times. The melody picked up again. When the song reached the end, I pushed in the stop. Grace was resting on the couch with her eyes closed. Time for bed, I motioned, raising my outstretched arms in completion of a big yawn. She smiled and nodded. I pulled her walker in close and helped her up. Before I got in bed, I checked on Grace one last time and asked if there was anything she needed.

She shook her head no. But there was something she needed, something we both needed—more time.

34

AN EARLY BEQUEST

On my last day, I got up early and petted Duke, who was asleep on the floor at the side of my bed. It would be a long drive to Chicago before finishing the trip the next day to Minnesota. On the way back, I would not have to worry about the unbearable summer heat of the South. I rented a reliable car with air conditioning.

I made my way to the bathroom, jumped in the shower, and felt the warm water sliding down my body as I cleaned up for the long car ride. After brushing my teeth and getting dressed, I quietly made my way through the house. Grace and I had talked the night before and she knew that I was not going to eat a large breakfast. I planned a glass of milk, a light meal to be alert for the initial drive.

To my surprise, Grace was already up and dressed. She was sitting at the dining room table. A glass of milk had already been poured. I smiled and said good morning, pulled out a chair and sat down. I picked up the glass and finished the milk. We looked at each other, not saying much.

When I looked in the direction of the antique music box, I noticed a large red bow fastened to its lid. She looked up at me and said, "You have to take it with you."

I told her I couldn't. The music box was your mother's. You enjoy it as much as I do.

"In my will, it is yours," Grace said.

"When the time comes, I will take great care of it," I said. Then I smiled, knowing what I had hoped for all along—that we were family.

Then she said, "But you have to take it now. It means more to me to see you enjoy it while I am alive than to know you will own it after

I'm dead. Of all the students who have lived with me, I'll miss you the most."

I had to catch my breath and swallow, so as not to choke. I looked at Grace with immense appreciation, and tears began streaming down my cheeks.

Then I became immensely sad. I was leaving. And to hear her mention a will, and a time when she would no longer be alive, dropped me to the floor. Both of us hugged each other and shed more tears.

I loaded the car with my books and clothes, and my lessons and my training, and my memories of the things I had to leave behind. There was one thing that I did not leave. Next to me, in the passenger seat, strapped behind the seat belt, was the antique, one-hundred-year-old Symphonia music box from Germany that once belonged to Grace's mother but was now keeping me company on the road home.

35

RETURNING TO CHICAGO

The drive home to Chicago was fifteen hours and included one stop at McDonald's for lunch, one stop at a gas station to fill the tank and empty my bladder, and one thirty-minute stop at an interstate rest station to take a short nap when I could no longer keep my eyes open.

Finally, I exited the highway and drove three miles through my old residential neighborhood. When I pulled in the driveway, my dad was there to greet me. He was working in the backyard while anticipating my return. He was all smiles and was happy to see me.

Earlier in the week, I called home and reminded him of the day that I was arriving. He surprised me. He said only rent the car to Chicago. Then he told me that he had found a used Volkswagen van that I could take to Minnesota.

Once parked, I emptied the rental car of my belongings including the antique music box, and he followed me into the house.

"Are you ready to drop off your rental car?" he said.

"Let's do it," I replied.

We followed each other in separate cars, he in his station wagon and me in the rental. After dropping off the car, I walked out of the shop and hopped in the passenger side across from my father. He looked forward and drove away from the curb. I looked over at him. I didn't know what to expect. My father was not a dad who hugged his adult children, at least not since my mother died. I had not been home since last summer. I had just received my diploma a month ago, a huge accomplishment, I thought. He did not make it to my graduation. I had not expected him to. Now that we were alone, I wanted to know what he was thinking. I wanted to know what he thought of me.

I was leaving for Minnesota in the morning and had no immediate plans of returning.

I desperately wanted his approval and, more important, his love. I needed to know that my hard work was worthy of recognition. But the ride home was as if nothing had changed between us. We talked about the weather. We talked about my drive from Alabama. He reminded me to get the brakes checked on the van when I reach Minnesota.

I got up early the next morning and checked out the van. It was spacious. The van had two seats, one for the driver and one for a passenger. The back of the van had been hulled out. It looked as if it had been inhabited by hippies who made a home of it more than drove it. When I put the key in the ignition and turned it, the engine started right away. To my surprise, it ran smoothly. What more could I ask for. I had transportation to Minnesota and a place to sleep while looking for an apartment.

I loaded the van with my clothes and books. I placed the music box in a larger box and surrounded it with towels to protect it. I strapped myself in with a rope across my lap because the seat belt was missing. As I backed down the driveway, my father came out and assisted with directions. Our driveway was narrow, and the van was wider than what I was used to driving. When I reached the street, I looked at him and waved. He rose his open hand high in the air. I shifted into drive and was off.

Halfway there, just north of Madison, Wisconsin, road crews were widening Interstate 90. In the left-hand lane, three eighteen wheelers followed one another closely, driving over the speed limit. Then all of a sudden, it was chaos. A cement truck leaving a construction site spilled wet cement on the road for normal traffic. I saw drivers in front of me frantically steering their vehicles to avoid a collision, but the trajectory of their momentum over the wet cement caused them to skid haphazardly. When the first eighteen-wheeler hit the wet cement, it skidded sideways and jackknifed across both lanes. The second truck veered to the left and safely made it into the median. The third truck, however, hit the second truck in the rear, and his trailer slid into my lane. No matter how hard I pumped the brakes, I kept sliding forward. When I finally stopped, the front end of my van was smashed in. The steering wheel pressing against my chest pinned me against the driver's seat. My knees were trapped below the dashboard. I was mentally shaken and my legs were burning. I looked down, and thankfully they were still there and I didn't see any blood.

I phoned home. My father sounded worried, but I told him that I was okay. He drove three hours north and met me at a hospital in Madison. X-rays of my legs didn't reveal any broken bones. The doctors assured me that everything was okay and released me that afternoon.

My father and I drove to the service station that towed the van from the accident. The van was totaled, but my music box was safe. I loaded my belongings into my father's station wagon and returned to Chicago.

Two days later, I flew to Minnesota. One of the doctors I would be working with picked me up at the airport and let me spend the week at his apartment until I found a place to live. After I did, my father drove to Minnesota and delivered the music box, a box spring and mattress, and some additional clothes. I asked if he wanted to spend the night with me in my studio apartment. Instead, he decided to make the seven-hour drive back home. I guess that a small apartment with no walls dividing us was a bit confining. Besides, there was only so much that we could say to each other about the weather.

PART IV

ANIMAL DOCTOR

36

THE FIRST FOUR

After three days of orientation and a day of shadowing the outgoing intern, whether I was ready or not, I was on the clinic floor with patients of my own. I thought about Grace and how she always encouraged me to do my best. Before I stepped into the hospital that morning, I made a promise to myself and to her that I would. Then I walked through the front doors.

My first case was a transfer from the overnight emergency service. A seventeen-year-old cat with chronic kidney failure, diabetes mellitus, and hyperthyroidism. He was admitted because of anorexia.

This thin scruffy cat looked its age. White hairs were interspersed throughout his black coat. His droopy eyes were dilated, and the corneas were hazy. When I approached his cage, he looked up, staring intensely at me as if he had the wisdom of an ancient Egyptian sphinx.

The admitting clinician from the overnight emergency service had done most of the diagnostic work and set up a treatment plan. Intravenous fluids trickled into a vein in the cat's leg to correct dehydration, and medication to block an overactive thyroid was prescribed.

Once hydrated, the cat's appetite returned. Eating and drinking made insulin administration and glucose monitoring more predictable. However, it was the veterinary student, a senior working with me on the case, who eased my concerns and allowed me the time to manage my other patients. She was smart, compassionate, and meticulous. She made precise adjustments in insulin as our cat's appetite increased. She decreased the fluid rate once dehydration was corrected. Our patient went home after a few days of hospitalization. The cat would never be cured of his chronic diseases, but now on medication and eating, he would remain stable for a long time.

I kept in touch with the student. After graduation, she continued her training and became a specialist in internal medicine. I knew she would. I recognized her abilities from our first meeting.

My second patient was a nine-year-old female miniature poodle. Missy's referring veterinarian called it in. He was frantic. He insisted that the university hospital see his patient right away. We obliged his request.

Missy, a white curly-haired poodle, weighed eight pounds. Her toenails were painted pink. She had pink ribbons attached to the hair on both ears. A month ago, Missy was diagnosed with heartworm disease. Heartworm is transmitted through the bite of an infected mosquito. The immature parasitic larvae travel in the bloodstream, and find their way to the heart, where they grow into full-size worms. The worms induce so much inflammation that they damage the heart and the lungs. If left untreated, dogs develop heart failure and die.

Medicinal arsenic is the treatment to kill heartworms in a dog. The medicine is not easy on the patient, and at the time that Missy was treated, the dose was much higher. Today, arsenical compounds to treat heartworm disease are safer and less toxic.

Missy received her first injection of the medication from her referring veterinarian. Within minutes, her legs buckled beneath her. She fell to the exam table and rolled over on her side. Her gums were gray, her breathing was shallow, and her pulses were barely palpable. Missy was in shock.

Knowing this, her veterinarian inserted an intravenous catheter and administered saline to improve her circulation and bring her blood pressure up. Corticosteroids were administered in case Missy was experiencing an allergic reaction to the medication. The veterinarian did not have the staff or equipment to monitor Missy's recovery and referred her.

Missy arrived in a cardboard box. Her owner babbled incoherent phrases of worry while gasping for breath so that she did not faint. When I peered in the box, Missy looked up at me. She was alert and her skin was pink. The intravenous catheter was still in her leg, and the fluid bag and the IV line were attached, but not running. Although weak for what was normally an energetic dog, Missy was no longer in immediate danger.

I asked if I could lift Missy out of her box and take a closer look at her.

"Yes," her owner said. "That's why I came."

To my surprise, I couldn't find anything out of the ordinary. Her breathing was quiet, her heart rate was regular, and her body temperature was normal. I had no clue as to why she collapsed. I took a blood sample and submitted it for analysis. All the values were normal.

New doctors tend to keep their patients in the hospital longer than what is needed. This is especially true when the reason for the illness is unknown. It takes a lot of experience to know *when to keep them and when to street them*, a wise doctor told me. As a new doctor, I held on to my patients for fear of discharging them too soon.

Even though Missy was stable and recovering quickly, I did not want to let her go home. I didn't know why she collapsed, and I wasn't sure if I was missing a serious problem. I asked the owner if I could hospitalize Missy for observation, and if she remained stable, I would send her home in the morning. The owner agreed, and my sense of uncertainty eased.

To my relief, Missy did wonderfully through the night. I discharged her the next morning without therapy. Still worried that I missed something critical, I persuaded the owner to come back in a week. I wanted to be confident that I had not missed diagnosing a serious disease.

When I examined Missy a week later, she was still the perfect picture of health. But her bloodwork was alarming. Her sodium was low, and her potassium was high, a hallmark of decreased adrenal gland function. With additional testing, the diagnosis was confirmed. Missy suffered from hypoadrenocorticism, an adrenal gland unable to respond to stress.

It was obvious why I missed the diagnosis the first time. When Missy collapsed, her primary veterinarian administered intravenous saline. Receiving fluids with sodium raised her blood levels of sodium, masking the disease. Receiving intravenous fluid flushed the high potassium out through her kidneys and into her urine. Treating her shock concealed her illness.

Hypoadrenocorticism is usually asymptomatic until the patient undergoes a stressful or fearful event. When stressed, the adrenal glands secrete corticosteroids. This endogenous drug ramps up metabolism and increases circulation, essentially waking up the body, preparing it for fight or flight. When Missy collapsed, she received an injection of corticosteroids, replacing what the adrenal glands would have released into her blood.

Missy made a complete recovery once I started replacement adrenal therapy. In fact, the owner remarked that Missy was a new dog, with energy that she had not seen since Missy was a puppy.

My third patient was Sam, a nine-year-old, eighty-pound yellow Labrador retriever. He was too weak to walk from the lobby to the exam room.

Sam's owner was an elderly man in his eighties, with thinning gray hair and glasses. His white canvas work pants and light-colored short-sleeve shirt loosely draped over his minuscule frame. Looking at the large size of his dog, I cannot imagine how the man made it in from the parking lot. But I was not going to have him struggle to get his dog into the exam room. I lifted Sam into my arms. With all eighty pounds of him pressed against my body, I felt a rhythmic thrill of a pronounced heart murmur vibrating against my chest. I placed Sam on the examination table, removed my stethoscope from my pocket, and listened to his heart. The murmur was loud. The pulses in his inner thighs were weak.

"Sam is tired all the time and drinks a lot," the old man tells me.

I answered back, "I think it is his heart."

I set Sam up for an ultrasound of his heart. I needed to know if it was a damaged heart valve or something more serious.

Later that afternoon, I got the result. Sam had a large mass on his heart. It filled the top chamber. His heart was struggling to circulate enough blood to the rest of his body.

Sam's owner had waited the entire day in the lobby for the results. I walked up front. I told him that Sam was stable. I explained the tests that we performed. Then I sat down next to him and told him the heartbreaking news. "Sam has a tumor in one of the chambers of his heart. There's not much I can do."

The man sank into the chair and his shoulder slumped forward. "How long will he live?" he asked me.

It is hard to predict, I told him. Maybe a week. Maybe several months.

He thanked me and said, "I just want to take him home."

I worried about Sam and his owner. I did not ask but somehow knew that this elderly man had no one else in his life but Sam. I brought Sam up front in a red wagon. When he saw his owner, he started wagging his tail. I transported Sam out to the car and gently lifted him into the back seat. I reassured Sam's owner that our hospital was open twenty-four hours a day if he needed our help for anything. He thanked me again and shook my hand, holding on to it longer than I expected.

I stood in the parking lot and watched as they drove away. And as they did, I remembered the monkey my father brought home for my brother and me. I remembered the veterinarian with red hair and large freckles who came to help when our monkey was sick. But mostly I remembered the veterinarian's kindness. How he was patient with the monkey and how the monkey trusted him. And when the veterinarian left, I remembered how sad I felt, knowing that the monkey was not going to live.

I stood watching the road after their car disappeared down the street. I wondered if I had spent enough time with Sam and his owner.

I wondered if he would need help getting his dog in the house. I wondered when Sam dies, and I thought that it would be soon, would his owner have enough compassion to get another dog. Not a dog to replace Sam but another dog to provide the company and love that is needed when you are alone. As I was alone when my mother died, and how having a dog made it easier.

My last patient arrived shortly after lunch. She was a black and tan, petite Yorkshire terrier, perfectly coiffed, big fluffy ears that overshadowed a thin face with a long delicate dark muzzle. The owner had a similar appearance. Perfectly coiffed big blonde hair over a thin face with a deep tan. Both middle-aged. Both worried. Both emotionally subdued.

"She will not eat," said the woman in a fearful voice.

She pushed a folder of papers for me to grab while holding the dog close to her chest.

I grabbed the folder and skimmed through the notes. The most recent information was on top and included lab data from a visit to her veterinarian that morning.

The owner followed me into an exam room tightly holding on to her dog. I offered her a seat while I continued to review the file. She sat down on the edge of the chair and looked up at me, waiting for an answer.

I looked down at her and said, "Her kidneys aren't working."

"How bad is it?" she asked.

Based on these numbers, I was very worried. Then I asked, "How long has your dog been sick?"

"Two days. She would not eat her dinner last night, and not her breakfast this morning. I saw several dried piles of vomit on the rug when I woke up this morning."

Acute forms of kidney damage are sometimes reversible, but they are also the most difficult to treat, and the prognosis is guarded.

I reached down to lift the dog from her arms. The owner hesitated at first and then finally handed her to me. I placed her on the towel that came with her on the exam table. I could tell that her dog was frightened. I asked the owner to come closer. Stand next to her and talk to her while I finish the exam. Having you present will make her feel more relaxed. Dehydration was the only physical abnormality detectable. After explaining that intravenous fluids and more tests were needed, I persuaded the owner to let me hospitalize her dog.

As I carried her down the hallway to ICU, everyone I passed smiled and remarked how cute she was. I smiled back without telling them how worried I was. To me, her laboratory data looked like antifreeze toxicity; her bicarbonate was low and so was her calcium.

When I got to the ICU, I handed the lab data to the clinician in charge of my service.

"Look over this for me and tell me what you think," I asked.

I did not want my past to control my decisions. But what happened next took me by surprise. He and another clinician in the ICU talked about the pathophysiology of the numbers. They discussed the anion gap, an acid-base condition, which in the face of kidney failure may have implications for an underlying cause. They talked about the chloride level in the blood. They had so many theories and so many questions that I wanted to know if they were more concerned about the data than the dog. Instead of modeling compassion, they played diagnostic *Jeopardy*. I imagined Alex Trebek reminding contestants to phrase their answers in the form of a question. Your next clue: "This sweet-tasting liquid is a common poison for committing suicide." What my supervising clinicians failed to grasp was that I had a dog in my arms that would likely die, and that I needed their help.

I moved to another side of the ICU and asked a technician to help me get an intravenous catheter in the front leg of my patient. The technician set out a catheter, white tape, a bag of fluids, and a fluid administration set. I shaved the fur over the vein on the dog's front leg. I tried inserting the catheter but was not having much luck. The first time the catheter went under the skin but alongside the vein. I tried redirecting it, but I could not get it to thread into the vessel. When I finally got in, a large hematoma appeared. Blood swelled under the skin around my puncture site. I could not get any blood back, and when I flushed saline in the catheter, the skin swelled around the entry site. I had blown the opportunity to use that vein. I pulled the catheter out and lightly bandaged the leg. I tried again. This time on the other leg. Again, I was unsuccessful. The veins on both forelimbs were now unusable. My patient was perfectly still during my attempts, but I noticed that her eyes were dilated, and her whiskers flicked back and forth. I didn't want to put her through any more discomfort. I blew out an exasperated breath of submission.

"I need a break," I told the technician. "Please set up a kennel for my patient."

As I left the room, I overheard my supervising clinician question my abilities, or my medicine, or my mental stability.

Some of his concerns were justified. I knew nothing about the anion gap. However, I knew that knowing everything about the anion gap was not going to help my patient.

Maybe I was unstable. Was it just a coincidence that on my first day as a clinician I would treat a dog with antifreeze poisoning? This déjà vu was beginning to feel like punishment. It was staring me in the face again. How many more times would I revisit my mother's suicide?

Enough, I told myself. I had a patient in there that needed my help. I returned to the ICU. I was able to insert an intravenous catheter into a vein in her back leg. I started intravenous fluids. However, the more I scrutinized her laboratory results, the more certain I became of the cause. At this stage of the game, she was going to die. I was sure of it.

By evening, my petite Yorkshire terrier had a seizure and then a second one. I talked to the owner and explained her dog's condition.

"She is no better, in fact, she is worse," I told her. "Her kidneys are shutting down. The antidote will not help. Her disease is too far advanced. There is nothing I can do to save her. I'm so sorry."

She thanked me for my care and then made the decision. "I want to euthanize my dog. I love her too much to watch her get any worse," she said.

How many more dogs would I have to treat with ethylene glycol toxicity? How many more times would I have to deliver gut-wrenching outcomes to clients? How many more times would I be forced to revisit my past? I was trained to ease the suffering of my patients. But could I take care of my own? Somehow, I needed to do more. I needed to figure out how to stop this from happening. Not only for mc but also for my patients.

37

AN OFFER

During my internship at the university, I learned that there were two types of people, those you were leery of and those you could trust. Carl Osborne was one I could trust.

Carl was a clinician in internal medicine. A true diagnostician with the curiosity of an archaeologist, he knew how to excavate meaningful data with extreme clarity and efficiency. And he had the brain of an enigmatologist: he knew how to put the pieces together to solve perplexing medical problems. Carl was in his fifties and wore large silver-colored, steel-framed glasses that covered most of his face. He combed his blonde hair from his forehead back and sported a short Amish beard. However, unlike the Amish, he had a matching mustache. He greeted me every day with a cheerful smile and a bright hello. He treated everyone that way. Talking to him one day, I was surprised to hear that at one time he was an overweight, heavy smoker. You could not tell from his current stature. He was thin and lively and traveled the world running marathons.

At the time, I didn't realize that he was so well known and revered as a clinician. He had a monthly column titled Poor Carl's Almanac in one of the trade magazines. He wrote pithy aphorisms to live by. They covered topics such as patience, endurance, friendship, and honesty. Some were quotes from the Bible: Faithful are the wounds of a friend, profuse are the kisses of an enemy (Proverbs 27:6). And some were his own creations. Friends don't coddle your weaknesses; they encourage your strengths. A wise person seeks to fix fault, not blame. And one of my favorites: *The reason a dog has so many friends is that he wags his tail instead of his tongue.* I was fortunate to make Carl's acquaintance. He was wise and kind.

During my internship, I gave a seminar on immune-mediated anemia in dogs. After the seminar, Carl approached me and asked, "How do you know when you know something?"

I never thought about it before. Our conversations were on so many levels, and I thought that he was searching for something profound. I was silent until he responded. "You know what you know when you can teach it to someone else." He did not stop there. "When is a fact a fact?" he continued.

I knew the answer to this one. "A fact is only a fact when you and everyone else agree to stop talking about it." I enjoyed our banter. He challenged me to think in ways that I had not thought about before.

When I had difficult clinical cases, I sought him out for advice. Sometimes his advice was directly helpful. And sometimes he sent me hunting with more questions than when I started. He taught me that just as a patient is an individual in health, my patients would be individuals in the expression of their diseases. Diagnoses would be similar but not as I read about them in textbooks. He taught me to use my scientific logic and my intuition. I will never forget the time he told me that I would always miss more for not looking than not knowing. Humbling, but true.

Years later, I would discover that Carl was also exceedingly kind. We were attending a veterinary continuing education meeting together in San Diego. We left the hotel and set out for a quiet dinner. On the way, we passed a homeless man begging for money. His clothes were soiled. His face was dirty and his hair disheveled. He said that he was hungry and asked if we could spare any change. The people ahead of us walked past and ignored the homeless man. If I had not been with Carl, I would have probably done the same. We did not. We listened to the man. Carl asked if he was hungry. When the man said yes, Carl asked if he could buy him dinner. The homeless man smiled, stood up, and came with us. We walked back to our hotel. Just before going in, the homeless man threw his sleeping bag behind several bushes to keep it safe. Carl escorted him inside and treated him to dinner at the fanciest restaurant in the hotel. The maître d'hôtel was not happy with our decision, but after he accepted a monetary tip, his disposition was in agreement with our plan.

I would like to think that Carl thought highly of me. I thought the world of him.

While still an intern, I was studying in one of the conference rooms near his office. It was past 7:00 p.m. Usually, I spent my evenings going over my patients' records and reading the literature about their diseases. That evening Carl came and stood in the doorway of the conference room. I looked up, smiled, and said hello. He did not immediately say hello back. Instead, he cocked his head slightly to the left and squinted his eyes as if he had something important or difficult to say.

"What do you plan on doing with your life?" he asked me.

"Before going to veterinary school, I was an electron microscopist in a cardiology research lab at the University of Chicago," I said. "I like research and was planning on being a pathologist."

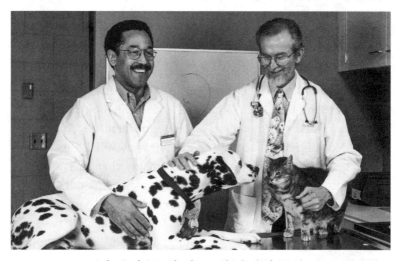

*Jody, Carl, Max the dog, and Adonis the cat in
University Veterinary Hospital, circa 2002.*

That started a whole new conversation on research. He told me that research training was learning how to ask the right questions and how to set up the right experiments.

"I agree," I told him.

Carl was silent for a minute and then he asked, "Would you like to do a residency in internal medicine with a PhD?"

I did not see that coming. A residency in veterinary internal medicine would require me to see patients and help clients. I enjoyed my internship but worried about my self-preservation working with distressed clients and sick animals for most of my life. I had a difficult time separating my happiness from my patient's success. I had an even more difficult time dealing with death, which was common with internal medicine cases at university hospitals. I looked up at Carl and slowly shook my head, *no*.

That was the end of our conversation. He turned around and left. I worried that I offended him.

A week later I would find out that my answer must not have been convincing enough. While I was working in the conference room late in the evening again, Carl paid me another visit.

"Jody, would you like to do a residency in internal medicine with a PhD?"

Before I could formulate a thoughtful reply, Carl told me that I needed to let him know soon because the University of Minnesota did not have an internal medicine position open and he needed time to create it and find the money to support it.

I was silent. I am always silent when I am not sure what to say or how to say it. His level of generosity was new to me. I was used to having the people I love manipulate me or hurt me. I was not accustomed to having someone, especially someone who hardly knew me, reach out to support me. Put me first. Invest in me. Put his resources into seeing me succeed. To avoid saying anything, I bit down on my lower lip and kept my mouth closed.

Maybe Carl saw something in me that I could not see in myself. Maybe I was not damaged as much as I thought.

This was the right thing to do and the right place to do it. He had given me something priceless, my confidence.

So I said yes. Yes, to being vulnerable. Yes, to trusting someone besides myself. Yes, to a worthwhile career caring for others. And yes, to a lifelong friendship with Carl Osborne.

But at the end of my internship, I had to question if the University of Minnesota was the right place for me.

After twelve months of hard work and sleepless nights, the interns and other house officers who completed their clinical training were awarded certificates. During the ceremony, pictures of us in action were projected on a screen while an emcee recapped the year with amusing quips and sometimes mishaps.

When it was my turn, they first showed a picture of the backside of my head with that of a black-haired poodle. The joke was about the style of my Afro matching the hair of my patients. Actually, the poodle's coiffure was a step up from mine. The poodle had been recently groomed. But when the emcee blurted out that I went to veterinary school to become a watermelon doctor, with those words he crossed the line. If the pain had not been so precise, I could have shrugged it off. When the audience laughed, I sank deep into my seat and retreated to the interior places I felt safe when I was a child.

I stayed for the residency and the PhD, but during that time I had a similar experience that taught me how ingrained bias and prejudice can become hardwired in the brain. I spent much of my time in the library. I used the space to think, research my thesis, and study for exams. The staff was helpful and interested in what I was accomplishing. I became friends with everyone who worked there. I listened to stories of their children, their parents, and their pets. But one day as I stood at the front desk to check out journals to take home, the main librarian made a remark that stopped me in my tracks.

"Jody, I don't consider you Black because you're not like them," she said.

I had to remind myself to not retaliate or stare. I was squinting as if my head hurt, and it did, so I quickly looked down. I leaned away from the counter. Without moving my feet, I felt as if I were sliding backward. Our faces and our friendship were now distorted. I didn't know what to think. Did she not see that I was Black? Did she think that Black men were incapable of education or insight or hard work? Was she trying to convey a compliment? Did she realize how painful that was to isolate me? Or was she clueless?

Weeks later she repeated herself, and then another time after that, "Jody, I don't consider you Black, because you're not like them." Each time I bit down on my lower lip. Each time I remained silent. Each time I disappeared without questioning her reasoning or her intent.

Melanie, a friend of mine, also worked in the library. Her desk was only a few feet away. When she heard those words, her blonde hair tossed backward. Her wire-rimmed glasses slid down her nose. Her eyes widened, and her cheeks filled with air. Then, her expression screamed at me, "Jody, why didn't you say something?"

I had no answer. I had no explanation. But somewhere deep inside I must have been returning to the night that my mother died. When my father smashed his wedding ring, threw it at her, and said get out of my life. And she did. I must have been remembering how words ignite conflict, conflict sparks action, and action leads to unintended consequences and misunderstanding.

Then my thoughts were interrupted. "Do you want me to talk to her?" Melanie grumbled.

I hesitated. I retreated. Doubt trounced reason. I told her no, it was okay. But it was not okay. I left the library and disappeared down the hallway. I needed time to cool off.

I thought about Grace Hooks and how Cornell University, after awarding her a full scholarship, refused to let her live on campus. I wondered what Grace would have done in my situation. That night when I got home, I called her. She said that I did the right thing. "If you are angry it will come off as anger." "Sometimes anger is good," she said, but not when you are with people you believe are kind deep within themselves. What you need to do is ask for clarification. Let her hear how idiotic her logic is. If she still does not get it, ask if you can reverse the roles. Put her in your shoes. How would she feel if you said *I do not consider you white because you are not like most of them.*

I never got to use Grace's advice. Melanie or someone else must have told her that her words were inappropriate. The librarian never apologized, but my alignment or misalignment with my race, or whatever race she thought I belonged to, was never mentioned again.

Carl Osborne knew that if given the opportunity I would stay after I completed my training. But at the time, the college was not hiring another internal medicine specialist. Nonetheless, he and I worked together to make it happen. With a focus on my research, he was able to construct a faculty position with extramural funding that included my salary. After completing my PhD in 1991, I took a job as an assistant professor in the College of Veterinary Medicine.

Carl was a strong advocate. He wanted more for me. He wanted me in a tenure-track appointment like the other faculty. He had another plan, to raise money for an endowed faculty position in my specialty. It would take two million dollars. He was willing to contribute the first half from his academic nest egg that he put together for research and graduate student training. He went to our department chair to get approval to raise the other million, but hit an unexpected roadblock. The chair had other plans for the department's future. That didn't stop Carl. He brought his plan up at the next department meeting. He was seeking approval to campaign for matching funds from corporate partners and the clients I served in the hospital. Departmental faculty was excited about his plan. However, when put to an official vote, he was blocked. The chair proclaimed that there was not a quorum to vote. This was odd. All previous departmental business was conducted without a glitch and I assume without a quorum. When departmental meeting minutes were distributed, the faculty consensus for Carl's plan was missing. In addition, the audiotape of the meeting supposedly broke just before the proposal was introduced. Carl did not take defeat lightly. We pushed forward anyway. When Carl or I lectured outside the university, we redirected payments to the campaign.

In 1998, the university was quoted in the newspaper, "If we had more minority scientists, we'd have more minority scientists." Based on those remarks, it was obvious that the university knew little about me, or my struggles to stay, and I was no longer quiet about it.

Shortly after the newspaper article, the university pledged bridging funds to support hiring underrepresented faculty. I applied and was offered a position at the veterinary college. But it was obvious that my college was not committed to hiring minority faculty. The college requested that I start my tenure clock at zero as if I were an inexperienced new faculty member. Accepting the job would wipe away recognition of my previous academic achievements even though I had already been promoted to associate professor and met all the requirements for tenure two years ago. I was not happy. They had just hired a veterinary cardiologist with three years toward tenure for working at a different university. I felt disadvantaged. These were my colleagues. I trusted leadership and assumed that they appreciated my hard work and loyalty. I was wrong, but this time I was not silent.

I took my crusade to the university president, explained my situation, and provided documentation to prove it. The university president never said that I had been treated unfairly, but he made sure that I was hired as an associate professor and would go up for tenure the following year. At the same time, he prevented my department chair and dean from interfering with the process. A year later, I received unanimous support for promotion and was awarded tenure without a hiccup.

In 2005, sufficient funds had been raised, and I accepted the offer for an endowed chair in nephrology and urology. By this time, I knew that the landscape for equity and fairness had improved. Or so I thought. The offer was low and below the salaries of recent hires in a similar position. I scratched my head in disbelief. I negotiated for equal pay. To my surprise, I was given a choice. Most would think that having a choice was an opportunity. This was not. I could take the original offer salary with a meager startup package or an equitable salary with no startup package. I took the equitable salary.

Were these offers strategic hiring, unconscious bias, or racism? Maybe all three. I will never know. What I knew was that the department's efforts were not entirely welcoming or program building. I should have been offered an equitable salary and an appropriate startup package like every other faculty appointment.

Then why did I stay? Cornell University offered me a faculty position more suited to my experience and expertise. I stayed at Minnesota because of my relationship with my adviser. Dr. Carl Osborne was supportive, trustworthy, collaborative, and creative, and we laughed together. As a team, we were focused and highly productive. He was my Grace Hooks of Minnesota.

38

VISITING GRACE

After moving from Alabama to Minnesota in 1984, I phoned Grace every week. I would tell her about work and my plans to visit at Christmas. I always referred to 1101 Bibb Street in Tuskegee as home. By the brief silence that followed, I knew that she was smiling and reminiscing. I was silent too. It was amazing how hearing each other's voices comforted us and transported us back in time as if we were still sitting around the dining room table eating dinner.

During my first year in Minnesota, spending Christmas with Grace was not possible. Every fourth night as interns, we worked a thirty-six-hour shift. There was a room near the front of the hospital with a bed and a desk. We were expected to sleep in the hospital in case an emergency arrived in the middle of the night. My day started at 8:00 a.m., taking in scheduled appointments. At 5:00 p.m. I moved to the emergency shift until 8:00 a.m. the next morning. The next morning was when I took care of the hospitalized patients I had admitted in the previous twenty-four hours. Coughing dogs needed transtracheal washes to search for a cause and cure for bronchitis or pneumonia. Icteric dogs needed an ultrasound or a liver biopsy. Dogs with suspected urinary cancer needed a bladder biopsy. Polyuric patients needed special blood tests to confirm adrenal or kidney disease. Patients who had swallowed rocks, fishhooks, corncobs, sewing needles, socks, pantyhose, or sharp chew toys needed an endoscopy to retrieve them, and if not successful the items were retrieved by surgery. Finally, after many hours one of my intern mates would start his or her thirty-six-hour shift, and I would get a chance to go home and sleep.

It was my luck of the draw that year. Christmas Day was assigned to me. I called Grace to let her know that I would miss not being there with her. But the following year when I accepted a residency position, I would do my best to ensure that I had Christmas off to fly back to Alabama and spend it with her. It took trading one of my days for two of another resident's, but I was not going to miss a second Christmas with Grace. After being away for more than a year, I boarded an airplane and rented a car. When Grace opened the door, it was as if nothing had changed. She stood in front of me with a wide grin, her gray shoulder-length hair parted on one side and combed back so that the curls rested behind her ears. She wore a floral apron with a loop around her neck and ties that fastened around her waist. Duke, her slightly overweight springer spaniel, was at her side. She reached her arms up and wrapped them around my neck. I bent my knees and wrapped my arms around her waist. I held on to her as I slowly walked her backward into the living room. We let go of each other, stepped apart, and looked at each other in the warm glow of the ceiling light. At first, not much was said. Her gaze went from my face all the way down to my shoes. Then she spoke, "I am so happy to see you, and you have lost some weight."

Grace sat on the couch, and I sat in the chair next to her. That was when I noticed that the antique Louis XV bombe vitrine curio cabinet with the collection of porcelain shoes was gone. I was sorry to see it go. The antiques were treasures collected by Grace's mother. These were the things that she had to remember her mother. But I also knew that Grace needed money to keep up the house and pay utilities. I did not ask about the cabinet's whereabouts. I didn't ask if she had to sell it. But I somehow wanted her to know that if she needed money that she could count on me. It was Christmas. I said nothing for fear of making Grace feel awkward. During my entire visit, she never brought it up either.

She wanted to know what it was like being a veterinarian. For the most part, I told her, I lose a lot of sleep. Being a new doctor, I worry about my patients. I want to do what is best for them. She smiled and patted me on the knee.

"I do not doubt that you are doing the best for them," Grace said. "Are you hungry?"

"Famished," I said.

"Let me make you a sandwich." Grace got up and headed for the kitchen. I saw that the dining room table was already set for Christmas dinner. Her mother's blue-and-gold-rimmed Noritake china dressed the table with linen napkins inside of silver napkin rings.

"I hope that you do not mind, but I order a precooked holiday meal from the supermarket," she said.

"No that's perfect. Less fuss and hopefully easier cleanup," I said. "Besides, you know why I am here. It is to be with you." She smiled as she brought in a ham sandwich and a cup of warm tea.

"I added a little sugar," she said, "just the way you like it."

I smiled back at her and took the tray of food. I was hungry and started eating. For the next five years, these were our Christmases. But in 1991 when I arrived, there was a change. When she opened the door, she looked tired. Her voice projected less audibly. Strands of her hair were loose. She still wore a floral apron looped around her neck and tied around her waist. She still smiled and reached up to greet me, encircling her arms around my neck. Duke was not at her side. She had called me earlier when he was sick. The diagnosis was lymphoma. He was old and the disease was advanced. She felt guilty for putting him down but would have felt even worse having to put him through treatment. I helped her make those decisions so that she would not have to handle them alone. I worried about her grief and her loneliness. When I phoned, she had a hard time talking about it. Although Grace had a large network of friends, I wasn't sure they could support her through the loss of her dog. Some may have not understood that losing a cherished pet is like losing a family member.

Grace and I walked inside and sat at our usual spots, she on the big couch and me in the comfortable chair. She kept rubbing her hands, the fingers of her right hand rhythmically stroking the palm of her left one. This time she didn't ask if I was hungry. The dining room table was not set for dinner. I asked if she ordered food from the supermarket for Christmas. I asked if I needed to pick up the food. She stared for a moment and thought about my question. Then she raised her hand to her mouth and behind it said that she was not sure but maybe she had forgotten to call them. I reassured her that I would drive to the store before it closes and I would cook the Christmas meal. It will not be as good as your cooking I told her.

She smiled.

While we were still sitting in the living room, Grace looked over her shoulder and into the dining room. She looked back at me and said, "Did you see the cat?" I didn't know what to say. There was no cat and never had been. In fact, I thought that Grace didn't like cats. That was the moment I knew that I was beginning to lose the person I loved so much. Grace's mind and independence were at stake. She needed my help.

39

MAUD

A year after completing my PhD, a time when I should have been celebrating my achievements and forging new opportunities, instead I
became critically aware of just how hopeless I had become, so much
so that I feared not only my incapacitation but that it might have a
fatal outcome. It was easy for me to work toward goals that others had
set for me, the joys of being a student. However, it was impossible for
me to set goals for myself, the responsibility of being a college professor. On top of that, I was lonely. My fears of intimacy and loss forced
me into isolation. All of my studying and research in preparation to
care for my patients was slowly being eroded by the realization that
I could not save my mother when all I had to do was tell someone,
anyone, that she was poisoning herself. I watched her do it to herself
and said nothing until it was too late. That was twenty-three years
ago, but last night it felt like it was yesterday. When I got up after a
restless night with little or no sleep, I had neither the strength nor
the courage to go to work for fear that what I was about to do or not
do could hurt my patients.

As the sun rose, I grabbed the edge of the blankets and slowly
pulled them up over my head, turned on my side, and retreated
into darkness for safety. I thought that I was alone. Then I felt Maud
scooch her back up against mine. I turned over and brought down
the covers. I looked at her and realized that at least one of us had a
good night's sleep. My thirty-pound, bright-eyed, energetic, wheaten
terrier extended all four of her legs in a wakeful stretch, pushing hard
against me. Annoyed at her exuberance, I looked down at her, this

time bringing my face closer, and narrowed my eyes to emphasize my disapproval. When I did, she ignored me and happily wagged her tail, extended her nose upward, and licked me in the mouth. She waited for me to get up and get out of bed. Lying there in such despair, I felt as if I were being swallowed up by my mattress, stuck like a fly caught in a Venus flytrap.

Maud held her gaze on my face, and her eyes widened as she patiently waited for a hand gesture, a blink, or some sign from me that I was getting up. I could not ignore her. "Okay," I grumbled. "I know you need to pee and eat. But I am not in the mood for *happy* this morning. Calm down," I told her.

She quickly stood up in bed and pounced onto my abdomen with her front paws. I winced in pain as I collapsed in the middle while my head and feet buoyed upward.

"Stop," I moaned. "Any more of this and you will crack one of my ribs."

Her enthusiasm was unstoppable. Maud jumped to the floor and ran to the kitchen. I peeled back the covers and pushed my way to the edge of the bed. My feet plopped to the floor. I sat there for a while, cupped my aching head in my hands, took in a long breath through my nose, and blew it out through pursed lips. I braced myself, stood up, and trudged down the hallway to the kitchen.

Maud scampered and turned in circles at the back door. Down, I wanted to tell her, but I just did not have the heart to break her joy because of my sadness. I opened the door and she ran out, squatted, peed, and galloped back up the stairs, taking two or three at a time until she was back in the house. She stood at my feet and again looked up at me.

"I know," I said. I opened a can of dog food, placed it in her dish, and set it on the floor. She gobbled up the food and licked the bottom of her dish until it was clean.

Maud and I shared something in common, a close brush with death. Unlike most dog lovers, who pick out an adorable puppy from a litter, bring it home, teach it to sit and stay, Maud was my patient before she was my dog. Yet it would have been great to have seen her as a puppy. Wheaten terriers start out as adorable reddish-brown balls of curly fur with black muzzles, large dark-brown eyes, and energetic, inquisitive personalities. As adults, they lose the brown fur and develop a silky coat the color of wheat. They don't shed, but require grooming every two to three months. If you see one in the show ring, wheatens have a long beard and a thick bang of fur covering their eyes. Maud's eyes were her best feature. That was how we communicated. They'd twinkle and jitter when she wanted me to play, throw her a ball and watch her scamper off to retrieve it. She'd intensely stare without blinking when she wanted what I was eating. That was annoying but effective. In the evening, her eyes would half close as she waited for me to finish my work and hop into bed with her. Whenever I sent her to the groomer, I sent along a note to remind them to clip the bangs and reveal her eyes.

Wheatens call Ireland their ancestral home. They are related to the Irish terrier and the Kerry blue terrier. Like other terriers, wheatens are intelligent working dogs, but unlike good working dogs, wheatens are not obedient and are considered untrustworthy. Maud was the opposite. She was exceedingly trustworthy, kind, and impeccably obedient.

I first met Maud when she appeared on my clinic schedule for leaking urine. Urinary incontinence is a common problem in younger and older large female dogs. At four years old and thirty pounds, Maud was neither.

During that first visit, it was easy for me to spot Maud and her owner in the lobby. She was the only wheaten. She sat on the floor and waited patiently, watching all the other dogs walk past. After approaching Maud and her owner, I introduced myself and ushered them into an exam room where it was quiet and where I could get to know them both. Maud's owner, a woman of average height in her late thirties with short light-brown hair and a mellow voice, energetically professed Maud's overwhelming glorious attributes. Maud was her prodigy child. Her enthusiasm was quite fascinating. I wanted to let her talk, but I also wanted to finish on time and not be late for my next appointment.

"Maud knew when I was pregnant," she said. "Not just with my first child but also the second, and the one I lost in between the two. She knew that my last one was a difficult pregnancy. I was bedridden for months. Maud stayed close to me the entire time. I was a wreck and constantly worried because I anticipated the worse. Maud remained as calm as a cucumber. When I became anxious, she was consoling. When I became sad, she snuggled into the bend of my arm or my knee and reassured me. When it was time for me to go to the hospital, Maud knew. She barked and wagged her tail with encouragement and then pouted as we closed the front door and left her home alone."

These stories were wonderful to hear but at first hard to believe.

Hearing Maud's uncanny ability to recognize the timing of her owner's parturition was amazing, but I also realized that I needed to stay on track with the appointment. I listened for an opportunity to interject and at the same time not negate her owner's joy of having such a wonderful companion. When I found an opening, I quickly interrupted. "I understand. With Maud spending so much time in your bed, leaking urine would be a huge problem for me too."

"Yes," she said. "I saw two veterinarians before you. Maud was prescribed a thyroid supplement and then estrogen to tighten her urinary sphincter, but neither of them worked."

Then I asked, "How long has Maud been incontinent?"

"Most of her life," she said.

Every time Maud heard me call her name, she slowly edged her way toward me until she was sitting at my side. Then she slowly placed one foot on the top of my shoe and leaned into the side of my leg, and I knew that we were going to be good friends. I told her owner that my patients rarely exhibit such affection for me.

"Maud likes you," she said. "There must be something special about you."

"I really care about my patients," I said. Then Maud looked up at me. I reached down and gently petted the fur on her head and whisked the hair from in front of her eyes.

Instead of lifting Maud on the table to finish the exam, I kneeled next to her and took a closer look while she stood next to me. She looked healthy, but the fur at the tip of her genitals was damp, a sign of urinary incontinence. When I was done, I stood up and asked if her previous doctors mentioned a disease called ectopic ureters.

"Yes, that is why I came to see you. You're the urinary specialist."

I chuckled, not because of what she said, but because of what she did not say. Too often, referring veterinarians affectionately referred to me as the *Pee God*. I was pleased to hear a more appropriate term for my medical acumen.

"What do we need to do next?" she asked.

"Can Maud come back tomorrow for tests? She will need a special X-ray to look for an ectopic ureter. We will need to sedate her for the procedure. Can I do a blood test today to check her kidney function?"

All was agreed. Maud returned the next morning. The outcome was no surprise. Maud had an ectopic ureter, a faulty connection of the tube that carries urine from the kidney to the urinary bladder. Instead of entering the urinary bladder, the ureter bypassed the bladder and entered more caudally into the urethra. Bypassing the urinary sphincter at the neck of the bladder prevented urine from being stored in the bladder. The anomaly was mild and difficult to detect, but it was obvious on the X-ray. Maud had surgery the following week and went home a dry, continent dog.

Wheaten terriers are also plagued with other inherited diseases. Like her distant relatives, Maud was diagnosed with kidney failure, mild but failure nonetheless. I told her owner, "We are fortunate to have caught it early. Only a diet change is needed, but I would like to see her every six months to make adjustments to her therapy when the time comes."

Like a trooper, Maud came in every six months. When she spotted me in the lobby, she'd rush to greet me, hop up on her back legs, and plant both front paws right in my abdomen. Her mom would apologize. I reassured her that no apology was needed. In fact, if Maud had not greeted me so affectionately, I would have worried that there was something wrong.

Maud continued to do well. Her kidney failure progressed, but slowly. Additional medications were not needed. When I saw Maud on my schedule for an unexpected visit, I became alarmed. I met them in the lobby. Maud greeted me as usual, full of enthusiasm. When she ran toward me, I braced myself so that she didn't knock me backward as her front paws pummeled my abdomen.

"How are you, girl," I said while briskly scratching behind her ears. Maude stretched her neck up, relishing the affection. After making our way into an exam room, Maud's owner told me that the family was moving to Texas.

"I am going to miss Maud," I told her.

Then she told me that they were not taking Maud.

"Why not?"

"Wheatens hate the heat," she said.

I agree, but there is . . .

"I want you to take her," she interrupted.

I balked at the idea. Instead, I asked, "How can you not take Maud with you?"

She repeated herself, "Wheaten terriers are miserable in hot weather."

I knew that she was right. Maud was an energetic snow bunny in the winter. She would lie on the ground with her bare belly flat against the snow enjoying the cool sensation. I tried to convince her that Maud would be fine in Texas, but her owner insisted that she wanted me to have her. I felt as if there were more to the situation than what the owner was revealing.

I tried to explain why I could not keep Maud. "I work long days. I would not want Maud to be isolated all day." I asked if she would be willing to donate her to the university clinic. I promised that I would find a great caring owner.

Those were not the words she wanted to hear. She was silent. In a low voice, she said, "Then I may have to euthanize her."

I became sick to my stomach. "Maud has a disease, but she has done incredibly well," I said. Then I told her that I could not be the one to euthanize her.

Tears began streaming down the owner's cheeks. She slowly knelt and picked up the end of Maud's leash from the floor. Without saying goodbye, she lightly tugged on the leash. Maud followed. They exited, and the door closed behind them.

The silence in the room felt eerie. Did I really hear that unless I take Maud she would be euthanized? I stood in a state of bewilderment and shame. Was Maud's owner telling me the truth? Her tears were real. Was her explanation real, because mine was not. I was now in direct confrontation with a dilemma and a lie. Not her lie, although her reasoning didn't seem to hold water. It was my lie that I was ashamed of. I could not take Maud because I did not know how long I could endure the pain of living. The death of my mother had weighed heavily on my conscience. I did not want the responsibility of caring for a dog to get in the way of my plans.

Two weeks later, Maud and her owner were back.

"I can't take her," I told her again. "Donate her and I will find her a good home."

"No," she said.

I can't euthanize Maud either. Not today.

As before, we parted in tears.

I wondered if Maud had any idea about what we were saying. I wondered how Maud felt about this.

When Maud and her owner called a third time, I relented. "If anyone should euthanize Maud it should be me," I said. I hope that Maud can forgive me, I told myself.

When they arrived at the clinic, I escorted Maud's owner to a private comfort room, and I walked Maud down the hallway to put an intravenous catheter in her front leg. To euthanize a dog you need a direct line to the heart. I needed to know that the euthanasia solution, once injected, would work quickly. Maud would fall into a permanent sleep within seconds.

As Maud and I walked side by side, I kept saying, I am sorry and you don't deserve this. Maud looked up at me seemingly unaware of the consequences that I dreaded. I lifted her up and gave her a tight hug before placing her on top of an exam table. A colleague came over to help. She knew that I was having trouble doing this.

I shaved a small patch of hair in the middle of Maud's forelimb. Maud kept looking at me and licking my nose. I slid the catheter into her vein and secured it in place with narrow strips of white medical tape. I covered the catheter with another bandage. I drew up the clear blue euthanasia solution into a syringe and stuffed it in the pocket of my lab coat. Maud and I walked back to the comfort room where her owner waited. She was sitting in a chair facing opposite from our entrance. When she turned around, her eyes were red and swollen. The tissue in her hand was pressed tightly over her mouth. She stood up and in an outburst of tears said, "I am donating her. Promise me that you will find her a good home."

"I promise," I said, as tears welled up in my eyes.

She reached down and hugged Maud for the last time. When she got up to leave, she said it again, "Promise me you will find her a good home."

"I promise."

I walked Maud to the back of the hospital to the dog kennels. I removed the catheter from her leg. I placed a bowl of fresh water and a small dish of kibble in the kennel. She climbed in as if nothing had transpired. She was energetic and happy as always.

Before heading home, I went to check on Maud. I opened the kennel door and sat on the ledge of the cage. Maud snuggled close to me. I petted her. She put her front paws in my lap and licked my hand.

"Okay, I am not letting you spend the night alone and in the dark," I said. I hooked a leash to her collar, and we walked home together.

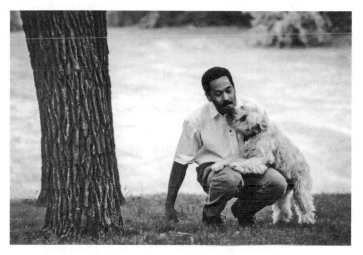

Maud and I play in a park in St. Paul, circa 1994.

After a month of living with me, I could not deny how special Maud was. That first night at home, I walked her to a rug on the kitchen floor and told her to stay. She looked up at me as if she knew exactly what I wanted. She quietly laid down, put her head between her two front legs, and resigned herself that this was her spot. When I woke up the next morning, she was where I had placed her. I was shocked but also felt guilty. I did not intend for her to be so obedient. After a week of sleeping in the kitchen, I moved her rug to my bedroom. When I turned out the lights, Maud quietly took her spot and laid down on the rug beside my bed. It was a treat to hear her snoring in the middle of the night. When I awakened in the morning, she was on the rug. After her morning walk and meal, she'd head back to the rug and wait for me to get ready for work. As I shaved and showered, Maud stretched out on her rug and patiently waited. Then we walked to work together. I was fortunate to have a job that eventually allowed pets.

A few weeks later, I heard a thump coming from the bedroom as I got out of the shower. I could not figure out what the noise was. Had a bird flown into the glass of my bedroom window? Maud was resting on the rug, undisturbed by the noise. It happened again the next morning. I was becoming concerned that maybe the plumbing in the house was faulty. By the end of the week, it was obvious. Each time that I got in the shower, Maud jumped into my bed, and each time she heard me turn off the water, she jumped back down onto the rug.

Her guile didn't stop there. After a few days, I didn't hear a thump. After my morning shower, I walked into the bedroom. Maud was stretched out over the bed with her head on my pillow. She looked up at me with an apologetic grin and a request to stay. I gave her a nod and briskly stroked my hand through the hair on the top of her head. The mystery was solved. The thumping noise was gone, Maud never slept on the floor again, and I never slept alone.

*

This morning was not the first time that Maud coaxed me out of a slump. I got out of bed, but this morning was particularly difficult. The day before, I performed a percutaneous liver biopsy on a jaundiced patient, and when I was done, the dog unexpectedly died. I will never know if it was my doing or the patient's disease, but I blamed myself. It didn't matter. The dog was dead, and it happened under my care and I felt responsible. I looked down at Maud. She looked up at me. I can't go to work today, I told her.

During hopeless times, eating ice cream helps me get through them. Häagen-Dazs rum raisin was the only flavor that eased the pain. I opened the freezer looking for a pint but remembered that I finished the last one in bed three nights ago. I closed the freezer and opened the refrigerator. Seeing the Reddi-wip on the door, I lifted the can, shook it, turned it upside down, and sprayed a generous portion of whipped cream in my hand. Without thinking, I quickly lapped it up. It was great, but I still felt sad. I dried my hand, walked back to the bedroom, crawled into bed, and pulled the covers over my head. I heard Maud's toenails clicking against the wood floor as she followed me. She stood at the entrance to the bedroom. At first, she was silent. Then she let go a muffled low bark. It sounded more like a cough. When I didn't move, she barked louder.

"I can't," I said. "Why don't you go without me?" I shouted. Maud stood there stunned. "I did not mean to scold you," I said. Then she jumped up on the bed and proceeded to dig into the covers with her forelegs. Her legs scurrying faster and faster. She bunched the covers into a heap, leaving me with none. She jumped back down to the floor and grabbed the corner of the blankets in her mouth. Then she stepped back toward the door, pulling at them as if in a tug-of-war. Finally, in one big scurry, with the blankets clenched between her teeth, she turned around and bolted for the door. When she entered into a gallop, the blankets slid off me and onto the floor. I knelt up in bed and faced her. She barked again while bouncing up and down on the blankets.

"Okay. I am getting up."

I went to the kitchen, turned on the cold water, and put my head under the faucet. I shook my head from side to side like a wet dog shaking off rain. I grabbed a towel from the counter to dry off. I got dressed, fastened Maud's leash to her collar, and we were off. She led the way, pulling me out of my sadness. We walked down Cleveland Avenue and then Gortner Avenue until we entered the University Veterinary Hospital and continued on a path to my office.

Everyone knew Maud.

"Hello Maud," said the receptionist, looking past the client that she was checking in.

"Hello Maud," said the custodian as he looked down from his ladder while he replaced a burned-out bulb in the ceiling. We kept walking, with Maud leading the way.

"Hello Maud," said the department secretary as we walked past the open door to the department office.

When we reached my office, Maud quietly sat and waited. I removed my keys from my pocket, opened the door, and we went in. I removed my white lab coat from the closet and picked up my stethoscope. Before I headed to the lobby to see my first patient, Maud looked up at me. I looked down at her and whispered, "Thank you for choosing me."

Even with Maud, there were still times that I suffered from severe loneliness, especially during my international trips. I agreed to a ten-city lecture tour in Spain during the Gulf War of 1990. Shortly after that, I lectured in Europe and Asia, usually for a week or longer. In many destinations, I required a translator. I did not speak their language, and they didn't speak mine. Having minimal communication, I felt more isolated than ever. I kept Maud in my thoughts. She provided me such happiness; I wanted to ensure her happiness too. I didn't want her to be abandoned if anything happened to me. I was careful. I always made sure that when I traveled locally or abroad, I left her with friends who would care for her in case I did not return, or fell off a cliff, or was found dead in my hotel room.

40

GREEN VOMIT

For many years, I taught a lecture called "Why Is This Dog's Vomit Green?" It was part of an elective course in urinary diseases for third-year veterinary students. I'd start the lecture by introducing the patient. (Do I tell this story because it is so personal? Because it may be, in fact, the core of my own life's trajectory? Do I say that Rocky was my most important patient, the one I so wanted to save, and the reason why?)

Rocky is an eight year-old stocky black Lab who carries his toys in his mouth when he goes on walks. Rocky is best friends with two young boys in a family who dress him up in their dad's old flannel shirt. Rocky does not mind: he basks in their playfulness. When the kids venture out, Rocky follows close. When they take a break on the floor, Rocky lies next to them, scooching his body up to theirs. They pet him, and when they do, he licks their faces.

Tonight, Rocky is sick. He is vomiting. Rocky's owner, the boys' father, brings him to our emergency room and tells us what is wrong. "Rocky was fine this afternoon," he starts. "We had a birthday party for one of the boys. Rocky, being his usual jolly self, began stealing their food, so we locked him in the garage. We wanted to give the kids a chance to eat. After the party, we brought Rocky back into the house. That's when he started vomiting. Rocky has vomited seven times. Mostly water at first and then foam. But each time, it was green. After he vomits, he drinks lots of water and he vomits again."

We examine Rocky. His pulse and respiratory rate are increased. We did not find anything else out of the ordinary.

The emergency veterinarian orders several tests. The blood phosphorus is up, and the bicarbonate is down. The X-ray of the abdomen is unremarkable.

Rocky is admitted. Intravenous fluids are delivered to correct dehydration. Antiemetics are injected under the skin to stop vomiting. He spends the night in our ICU.

The next morning, Rocky is transferred to the internal medicine service. Rocky's new clinician sees me walking down the hallway. She hands me the laboratory data and asks, "Why is this dog's vomit green?" I stop, look over the lab data, and bite down on my lip. I look up at her and tell her that I am very worried.

Now that I have piqued the interest of my student audience, I stop presenting the case. I leave the lab data up on the screen for the students to continue to mull over the results and ask, "Can you solve the case of the green vomit?"

I want the students to think through the problem. I pass out blank index cards for them to write down their thoughts. Here are several questions to help guide you: "What disease is likely, and what test would you order next?"

I give them time to think. I also give myself time to let go of the anxiety that builds up in me every time I start this lecture.

Of course, I know why Rocky is vomiting. I knew the instant I was handed his laboratory data. Rocky ingested antifreeze, the same poison my mother drank to commit suicide. Recalling my mother's death fills me with my familiar sadness. I turn away from my students and face the screen. I do not want them to see the vulnerability on my face. It takes me a few minutes to collect my composure before I can continue.

"Hand in your answers," I announce.

Some ask for more time.

"Okay, but no more than a few minutes," I say.

As I collect the cards, I look over their answers. I am not surprised that I have not come across a correct response yet. I do not tell them that, but instead, remind them that real life is a hard teacher . . . Mother Nature gives the test first, and the lesson later.

After collecting all the cards, I enthusiastically announce, "Let's start the lesson." I write the topic on the board, Diagnosing Common Kidney Toxins. I hear several groans from the class. I realize that they probably thought that Rocky is vomiting because he ate a rubber ball or corncob.

I draw a line through the topic. Then in capital letters I write, MEMORIZE THE SIGNS OF ANTIFREEZE TOXICITY. One student in the back of the room shouts out, "I knew it."

I ask them, "Why did I change the topic?" After a short pause, I answer my own question. "Because although there are many toxins that damage the kidneys, antifreeze has the shortest window of opportunity. You must react quickly. Therefore, memorize the clinical signs of the disease. You have a short time to make the diagnosis, administer therapy, and save the patient. It is not easy saving dogs that have ingested antifreeze. Even if the dog survives, your patient will likely have permanent kidney damage.

A student up front raises her hand, "What made you think it was antifreeze?"

Her question catches me by surprise. I pause and lean against the desk for support. I debate telling them that when I was nine years old my mother committed suicide by drinking antifreeze. But I do not. I push myself up from the desk and stand up straight. I repeat the question. "What made me think that Rocky drank antifreeze? Let's put the clues together."

The principal component of antifreeze is ethylene glycol. This small molecule irritates the stomach, causing Rocky to vomit. As the toxin is further metabolized, failing kidneys will cause vomiting.

Most antifreeze contains sodium fluorescein, which is green. Fluorescein is added to antifreeze to help car mechanics spot any leaks in the car's coolant system. Hence, the green vomit. When you shine a black light on it, it fluoresces.

Many antifreeze solutions also contain phosphorus rust inhibitors. As extra phosphorus is absorbed, the phosphorus concentration in the blood goes up. In the later stages of antifreeze toxicity, the phosphorus goes up because the kidneys fail to remove it from the blood.

Lastly, ethylene glycol is metabolized by the liver into several organic acids. The body gets rid of some acids through the lungs. This explains his increased respiratory rate. Rocky is trying to blow the acids out of his body. Acids are also buffered by bicarbonate, which explains the low concentration of bicarbonate in the blood.

You may wonder how Rocky got into the antifreeze. Rocky's family kept antifreeze in the garage on a lower shelf. I guess that Rocky was bored, locked in the garage. He chewed the container and lapped up the chemical. Antifreeze has a sweet taste. Rocky must have concluded that the antifreeze was a good alternative to his food and water.

Another student asks, "Does Rocky die?"

The air escapes my lungs in a despondent "Yes, Rocky dies." By the time Rocky's illness was diagnosed, it was already too late. We were past the window of opportunity. The poison had been in his body for more than twelve hours. The damage to his kidneys would be severe. Intravenous fluids, peritoneal dialysis, and antiemetics would not reverse the inevitable. "Rocky was euthanized four days after the diagnosis."

"Not all cases end this way," I tell the students. "There is an antidote."

Antifreeze is not toxic. The breakdown products of antifreeze are the culprits. They damage the kidneys and other vital organs. If we can block the metabolism of ethylene glycol long enough to permit its excretion, or remove the toxin with hemodialysis, the dog is saved.

One medication that can block the breakdown of ethylene glycol is 4-methylpyrazole. To be effective, you must administer it early. If the antidote is not available, strong whisky is a reliable substitute.

The enzyme that breaks down ethylene glycol is the same one

that breaks down alcohol. If you get the dog drunk and saturate this enzyme, there will not be any left to break down ethylene glycol.

I feel my stomach heave. It presses hard on the side of my abdomen. I am sure that the students can tell something is wrong by the shallowness of my voice. I tense my abdomen and keep lecturing.

"A winter ritual in Minnesota is closing down the lake cabin. Antifreeze is poured into the toilet to prevent the plumbing from freezing. In the spring, it poses a threat. The five-hour car ride north to open the cabin is a joyous trek for the family and their dog, but perhaps too long a ride for a happy-go-lucky dog to endure without water. When they arrive and open the cabin, a smart dog will remember its way to the toilet to quench its thirst. Initially, it may go unrecognized that their beloved dog just drank antifreeze. It may go unrecognized for hours. When they figure out what happened, they need to get their dog to a veterinarian quickly. Remember your window of opportunity is short. The ride back may be far, and every minute counts. As the chemical is broken down into its toxic end products, the process needs to be stopped early if you are to save the dog. Instruct the owners to find a liquor store. There are always more liquor stores than veterinary clinics. When they find a liquor store, tell them to get their dog drunk. Put vodka in bread or anything that the dog will eat. Alcohol dehydrogenase is one hundred times more likely to become preoccupied with vodka and leave the ethylene glycol alone. Managing a drunk dog is much better than managing a dead dog."

It is difficult to stay in the lesson with such strong feelings pulling me back. The ultimate irony—if only my mother had gotten drunk. If she had, maybe she would be alive today. But that was not her first suicide attempt. Even if we got past that January 2, there would have been another one, another day, and another poison. But what of the alternative? If she had survived, maybe she would have gotten the help she desperately needed to stay alive?

"Time's up," I announce. I end the class a little earlier than usual. That's enough for today. "We can discuss other kidney toxins tomorrow."

I stand mentally off-balance, watching students file out. When the last student reaches the door, she turns around and says, "I will see you tomorrow, Dr. Lulich."

I half-smile, recognizing her concern. "Yes, see you tomorrow."

I teach this class every year. And each year I think that it's going to get easier. In some ways it does: I see what's coming and adjust sooner. And in some ways, the teaching is more difficult; I do not know exactly when my emotions are going to grab me by the guts. But each time I teach, it is different. What frightens me most are the times I unknowingly hold my breath. I am not aware that I am in trouble until suddenly I gasp for air. It is as if someone were holding me underwater and at the last minute pulls me up to the surface to breathe. I was too late to save my mother, but I know that if I teach this lesson, and my students learn it, many animals will be saved.

PART V

———

LETTING
THE
LIGHT
IN

41

MISSING GRACE

Janet called me. "It's time," she said.

Janet, like me, had lived with Grace while attending Tuskegee University. Like me, Grace was a second mother to Janet. We both agreed to help Grace when she could no longer take care of herself. Unlike me, and fortunately for Grace, Janet lived in town. We both knew that one day Grace might not be able to take care of herself. We knew how much she appreciated her home and her independence. We wanted to keep her in her house and around the things she loved for as long as possible.

When Janet said that it was time, I knew what she was referring to. After I left to live in Minnesota, other students lived with Grace. They provided company and, by paying a modest rent, helped Grace pay utility bills. However, over time, Grace's mental abilities began to deteriorate.

The night that Janet called, Grace had phoned the police and reported a man lying on the floor in her dining room. She told the operator that the man was dead. When the police arrived, there was nobody on the dining room floor. Grace had hallucinated the incident. I cannot imagine how she conjured up such an image in her head. I was worried. Was this a recollection or an evocation? Had a man actually died in the dining room? If not in this house, maybe a previous house. Was this a family secret? When her stepfather died, where did she find him? On the dining room floor?

I could not have imagined how frightened Grace might have been. I was grateful that Janet was there to help. She made all the arrangements. She moved Grace to Magnolia Haven, a nursing home on the edge of town, and closed up her house.

I visited twice a year. I had never visited a nursing home before. There were white walls and white linoleum floor tile with streaks of gray. The staff wore white. The desk where I checked in was white. It was a sterile environment compared with Grace's intricate home.

The residents were in wheelchairs. Some were being pushed by the staff to the dining hall or back to their rooms. Others maneuvered their chairs with their feet. They'd reach out with the heel of their shoe and pull the chair forward. It never went straight, but it was an exercise to keep them going. I wondered if this was what the end of life is supposed to look like.

After checking in, I headed to Grace's room. On my way, I recognized one of the past deans of the veterinary school. He was strapped in his wheelchair. His head slumped forward and his chin rested on his chest. I knelt in front and reintroduced myself.

"Hi. I graduated from Tuskegee's veterinary school many years ago." He could barely lift his head. His eyes began to focus in my direction. I was not sure that he heard me. I said it again. "Hi, I graduated from Tuskegee in 1984." His eyelids lifted. Once his eyes met mine, he smiled. I smiled back.

"How are you? Do you need anything?" I said. He was silent. His head hovered and then lifted slightly. I waited a few moments. His eyelids slowly lowered and then his head sunk back down. He never said a word. I gave him a gentle pat on the side of his leg. "I am going to visit a friend. I will come back and say hello on my way out," I said.

I got up and headed down the hallway. When I reached Grace's room, I stuck my head around the door and peered into the room. I wanted to surprise her. The newspaper was in her hand, but her eyes were closed. I stepped all the way in, and when I got close, I enthusiastically said "Grace." Her head lifted and her eyes opened. She formed an enormous grin. In a soft voice, she said "Jody," and then let out a soft joyful sigh. We spent the afternoon catching up. She could not remember where I lived. However, she remembered her dog, Duke, and the night that he escaped out of the yard. That she woke me up in the middle of the night to help her look for him. I told her that I was teaching veterinary students at Tuskegee this week and that I would be back every afternoon while here. She smiled again.

Over the years, her memory and health aged rapidly, but she always smiled when I entered her room. She always recognized my face, but she did not always say my name.

Janet and I kept Grace's house as she had it, with the hope that one day Grace would be able to come back if we could find a suitable service to care for her at home. Maybe Janet hoped that I would return to Tuskegee to teach and live in the house and take care of Grace.

When it became obvious that neither of those options was going to happen, Janet and I made plans to categorize and photograph the items in Grace's house and put them up for sale. I told her that I could sell them online. It would bring in additional cash to help pay for her care. She agreed. Within the month, I made a trip to Tuskegee.

On an early afternoon in March, the sky was clear, the sun was bright, and the breeze was cool. Good for us because the electricity had been turned off years ago. We depended on the afternoon light to work. Janet unlocked the door, and we walked in. The house was as I remembered it, except for the new musty smell of old books. Old books do not fare well closed up in a dark, warm house. On my right, a comfortable chair was perched against the wall where the Louis XV curio originally stood with its collection of fine antique porcelain shoes. In front of me was the secretary with serpentine drawers. On my left, the fireplace. On the mantel sat the gilt spelter music box with the clock. Above the mantel, a picture of Tuskegee woods in pastels hung on the wall. Gazing around the room, I saw the textured beige couch where Grace sat during our first meeting. I peered in the den and smiled, remembering that every night we watched the ten o'clock news. Like clockwork, Grace would fall asleep as soon as the weatherman came on with his USA map of temperatures on the continent. I kept walking straight until I reached Grace's bedroom. A collection of ceramic elephants relaxed on the nightstand. I always wondered why she collected them. Next to the nightstand was the low lady-slipper chair that she sat in when I braided her hair.

Janet asked if there was anything that I wanted. I looked at the high-back Jacobean chair in the dining room. Grace's mother had pulled that chair from the garbage at nearby Huntingdon College, which had no use for it during a remodel after a fire. Grace would sit in that chair, read the mail, and sometimes take an afternoon nap. She looked relaxed in that chair, yet the chair was so large compared with Grace's small form that it made her look humble and regal at the same time.

There was another item I wanted, the dining room light fixture. A brass chandelier with four small lion heads equally spaced around a central orb. In the mouth of each lion was a brass ring that dangled each light and glass globe. The chandelier bathed us in a warm yellow glow as we ate dinner together. In that dining room, we talked about our day and solved the world's problems, which were mostly our own. It seemed odd to become attached to a ceiling light fixture, but it was more about the way that fixture illuminated our faces. How it cast shadows over our hands. And how I watched Grace's shadow leap across the dining room walls as she cleared dishes from the table and took them into the kitchen. Janet agreed, and I had the items shipped to my home in Minnesota.

Next, I took pictures of the fine dishes and their serial numbers on the bottom. A Dresden compote, a Spode platter, a bisque boy and girl on a swing. Some items were beautiful but had little value, and some were old and worth thousands. I took pictures of the cabinets, the large mirror hanging over the dining room buffet, the Sheraton table, the silver teapot service, and the Italian pottery.

I returned to Minnesota and posted several of the items online. The bisque boy and girl on a swing sold instantly. Janet returned to the house to collect it to ship to its new owners. She walked in and saw papers strewn over the floor. That was not how we left the house. The Sheraton-style mahogany table and its four Regency chairs, the large mirror with the ornate scalloped wood frame, and the buffet that rested against the wall were gone. Fine china was missing, as was the large Spode platter from England, the pictures from the walls, the antique clock from the mantel, and a very old Chinese lamp from the side table. Janet ran to the back door and shrieked. The lock had been broken. Many of Grace's valuable possessions were stolen. Hearing this, I felt as if they had been taken from me.

Janet and I decided that we could not wait to sell the items online. I contacted a dealer and flew back to Tuskegee. The dealer met me at the property and sold the remaining items for a little over two thousand dollars, a fraction of their value, but it was better than letting thieves take them. We never told Grace that the antiques that her mother collected over many years were stolen and that we needed to sell the others.

And within a year, Grace would be gone too. She spent most of her final days sleeping; gradually she stopped eating. She responded little to my touch and my voice. We hoped that providing nutrients and water through a feeding tube would revive her enough to help us discuss end-of-life decisions. It did not. On April 23, 2001, Grace, at the age of ninety, died.

As stipulated in her will, her body was donated to science. It was shipped to the medical center in Birmingham, Alabama, to help train medical students.

Years later, I discovered that after serving medical students, her body was cremated. Louis, one of the students who had lived with Grace before me, received her ashes.

I didn't know Louis, but I wanted to ask him if I could have her ashes. I introduced myself over the phone and explained that I also lived with Grace while I attended Tuskegee. Through our conversation, I kept wondering what he had planned for her ashes. I thought that maybe Grace requested him to scatter them over a beloved location, Grace's childhood home, or her grandmother's grave in Poughkeepsie, New York. Finally, I asked, "Do you have Grace's ashes?"

"Yes," he said.

I was silent. Relieved but silent. I didn't know how to ask for them. I asked Louis if he knew that Grace attended Cornell University. Then

I told him how much Grace wanted to be a part of college life and how much she fought to live on campus. I told him that I wanted to put her ashes in a place that she deserved but was denied. He agreed and thanked me for caring so much for Grace.

I breathed a sigh of relief. The ashes arrived by Federal Express at my home in Minnesota. I bought an airline ticket to Ithaca, New York, with a stop in Atlanta on the route home.

On a sunny spring morning, I stood on the front lawn of Sage Hall, a dormitory built in 1875 to house women students attending Cornell University. Between 1926 and 1930, Grace and other female African American students were denied campus housing because of their race. The building was just as Grace had described it. Sitting on top of a small grassy hill was an impressive crimson-red brick building with a witch's tower in the center above its entrance. The tower was capped by a steep pointed black roof. As I looked up, I imagined Grace feeling unwanted and angry, and became angry myself. She not only suffered an appendicitis attack requiring surgery but also had to look beyond the racism and focus on her education during her years at Cornell.

Grace also described a peaceful meandering creek behind Sage Hall. I walked around the building, imagining a wide-eyed Grace wanting to be a part of college life. It was ironic to learn that Henry Sage provided the construction endowment to attract and retain female students.

Today Sage Hall is no longer a woman's dormitory. Restoration in 1998 transformed the century-old building to house the Graduate School of Management, but the meandering creek that Grace talked about behind the building was still there. I sat down on one of the benches at the edge of the creek and emptied the sack containing half of Grace's ashes. The ashes spilled between blades of grass and tumbled down the bank. A strong wind buffeted against my body and at the same time collected some of Grace's ashes and spread them over the sidewalk, up the street, and down into the creek. At first, I wished that I had dug a hole and secured them to the spot. Then I realized that Grace had walked all over this beautiful campus. Her ashes were going to those places that brought her honor and anguish.

The next day I got back on the plane. My next stop was Georgia. In Atlanta, a high school friend met me at the airport. I stayed at her house that night. The next morning we drove to Tuskegee. I gave a lecture at the veterinary college in the morning and met Janet at Greenwood Cemetery on Old Montgomery Highway at noon. Janet and I hugged, and then she led the way to the burial site of Grace's mother and stepfather. One wide headstone with the names and dates of Grace's mother, her stepfather, and Grace were etched in the stone. Grace's name was only a marker indicating her passing. Her body was never buried here. I assume that when Grace's mother planned the site, she didn't know of Grace's end-of-life plans. I pulled the other half of Grace's ashes and a small garden spade out of my backpack. I handed the ashes to Janet, and she took a closer look. Fine gray dust moved from side to side as she inspected them through the clear plastic bag. I knelt and dug a small hole in front of Grace's tombstone. The ground was hard, the dirt dry. There were no trees in the cemetery, only grass, and orderly arranged headstones. Janet handed back the plastic bag. I opened the top and gently poured Grace's ashes down the hole and filled it with topsoil to keep her safe.

Before heading back to Atlanta, we drove past the old house at 1101 Bibb Street. Two men in their thirties were sitting on the front porch talking so loudly that one would assume they were arguing. When I slowed down and looked up, they stopped and looked in our direction. I wondered if they had any idea of the history of that house and who lived there before them. I noticed hundreds of tiny pine cones in the front yard and over the steps from the two tall pine trees flanking the porch. I imagined the crunching sound they made, squashing them under my feet as I walked up those steps the first time that I met Grace with her dog, Duke, in 1980. What a wonderful time in my life, I thought. I am going to miss you Grace, I whispered. Then our car sped up, and we drove back to Atlanta. I could not stop thinking about my time in Alabama during my plane ride home.

42

ANOTHER LOSS

In June 1998, in the middle of the afternoon, the phone in my office rang. I recognized the caller ID. My father was calling from Chicago. I picked up the phone. I heard him breathing heavily and then stuttering. "Dad," I said. Before I could ask what was wrong, he began to sob.

Thelma had been with my father for twenty-six years, almost twice as long as he was married to my mother. I was pleased that it lasted so long. My father was argumentative. For the sake of a challenge, he would defend a viewpoint in opposition to his beliefs. Thelma, on the other hand, was a pacifier. She would lie to keep the peace, but she also knew when to stand her ground. When she saw my father spending too much leisure time with a tenant, she bluntly reminded him that there was no sex worth five hundred thousand dollars, which was close to half of the value of the property they shared. Others would describe their relationship as mutual codependency. One neighbor summarized it perfectly: "Your father would throw a brick through the window of a hearse on its way to the cemetery and hide behind Thelma, who would smooth out the rough spots."

Through tears, he told me that Thelma was dead. The words astounded me. It took me a while to respond, and when I did, I said how sorry I was. "I am going to miss her. I am sorry that I am not there with you. What can I do?" I asked.

He told me that the funeral was next week and asked if I was coming home. He explained that her death happened quickly. He was so upset and not sure what happened. "Her sister took her to the emergency room two days ago," he said. "Thelma collapsed. She was in shock. Her heart was weak. I told her not to eat all that junk food."

I had not been to a funeral in thirty-two years, not since my mother died. Thelma was important to both of us, and my father needed me. I decided that it was time for me to change.

On the day of Thelma's funeral, I took an early morning flight to Chicago. I wanted to arrive before anyone else. When I saw the white enameled casket up front, I knew that my father had nothing to do with the funeral. I later discovered that Thelma's sister Wardine made all the arrangements. My father would have chosen a simple ceremony with a wood casket.

I looked across the room. There were four other people in the hall when I arrived. The casket was open. I walked up and looked in. Thelma was being buried with her glasses. How considerate, I thought, but also ironic, since her eyes were closed. While I stood there, memories of my mother washed over me. I was that nine-year-old child again, alone and at a loss as to what I was supposed to do with my life. I shook my head, because I was doing what I wanted to do with my life.

Before I took a seat there was one thing that I wanted to do ever since my mother died. I slowly took my hand out of my pocket and slid it up alongside the casket. I rested my hand on the edge of the opening. I looked around, and no one else was near. After mustering up enough courage, I reached in and touched Thelma's hand. I was expecting it to feel smooth and pliable. It was not. It was cold and leathery. My sadness vanished. This was Thelma's body, I thought, but it was without her kindness and her generosity. It was without her humility and her silliness. It was without her strength and her patience. It was without her laughter.

I took a seat, three rows back on the left. The seating quickly filled in. Thelma was popular and liked by many. Wardine sat up front in the middle. My father changed his position often. Sometimes sitting and sometimes standing. At the end of the ceremony, I caught up with him. He was more upset than sad. He blamed it on her diet and the piece of chocolate cake she ate the night before going to the hospital. I felt tremendously sad for him. I was returning to Minnesota on a flight later that evening. I hugged my father. He was still so upset that he didn't hug me back. I felt sad because my father would be going home alone.

The following week I called home. "Dad, would you like to move to Minnesota?" I told him that Minnesota winters were hardly different from Chicago's. I told him that for the value of his home, he could easily buy another one in Minnesota and have money left over. I told him that if he moved I would be closer and could care for him with anything that he might need.

"What about your brother, Gary?" my father asked.

I did not tell my father that I still didn't feel safe around Gary. I didn't want Gary living that close to me. I paused and changed my mind. I reassured my father that Minnesota was only a short plane ride away. If you should need anything, I can be there in a couple of hours. I will come whenever you ask.

43

PARENTING

Now that Thelma was gone, I hardly went home to Chicago anymore. My father and I developed a closer relationship, but this happened over the telephone. So when he calls and asks if I could speak to my brother, I did not know what to say. The way he said it, I sensed that he wants me to be the parent again. I remind myself that I need to develop better boundaries when it comes to our dysfunctional family.

The relationship between my father and brother has always been one of codependency and manipulation. When Gary and I were younger, he was the one with superior intelligence and opportunity. His IQ test scores were off the scale. The school wanted to send him to centers for high achievers and specialized training. When our mother died, Gary's world collapsed around him. He no longer had the desire to excel. Instead, he became quite adroit at blaming others for his difficulties. Instead of allowing my brother to find a way out, my father enabled him. Gary does not graduate from high school. He never holds a job. He never develops life skills or the self-esteem that comes with hard work and accomplishment. To make my brother happy or maybe out of parental guilt, my father supports him. When he becomes an adult, my father purchases a house for him and gives him money when he needs it. After Thelma dies, my father sells Gary's house, maybe for the money or maybe out of fear of being alone. This forces my brother to move back home with him.

My father hands my brother the telephone. I hear his voice in the background telling Gary that your brother wants to talk to you. Before I say a word, my brother says, you know that Dad thinks that you are wasting your life.

What do you mean? I said.

Dad says that doctors like you do nothing but kill your patients. Instead of using nutrition, you put chemicals in their bodies. You harm your patients and make them sicker.

I take in a breath and try not to explode. Here I am working hard to please my father, and my brother tells me that I am having the opposite effect. I also realize that my brother is cruel. When he was in high school, he decided to make money by breeding Doberman pinschers and selling them. Our backyard had as many as eleven dogs barking and stepping in their own feces. The neighbors threatened to call the Humane Society on us if we didn't clean up the mess. To teach the dogs to not pick up any poisoned food tossed in the backyard, my brother put an electrical wire in a slice of hot dog. Every time one of the dogs reached for the treat, they got shocked and dropped it. The dogs quickly learned to only accept food that came in their bowls. But when one of the dogs kept attacking the others, my brother turned vicious. He kicked the dog as hard as he could. Once he put a noose around its neck, hanging it from a rafter in the garage so that only its back legs touched the floor. Only when the dog was too tired to stand on its back legs did he untie it. It was his way of breaking the dog in, he'd say. I could no longer tolerate his cruel training tactics. I felt sorry for the dogs and worked hard to make sure that they found homes as quickly as possible.

My brother was getting even with me by telling me what my father thought about my work. I knew that Gary was telling the truth. I overheard my father on the phone say those exact words, not about me but to a friend in the hospital. He warned the man that the best thing he could do was to leave the hospital and to do it before his doctor killed him.

"I know, Gary," I said. "I'm okay with it." However, I was not okay. I wanted my father to be proud of me. I tell Gary that Dad needs your help to get a few things done around the house. I tell him that sometimes, Dad asks for help because he is lonely and wants your company. Put Dad back on for me, I tell my brother.

"Hi, Dad. I talked to Gary, but I cannot keep doing this. You and Gary need to straighten this out for yourselves. If he is not going to help you, hire someone else."

After I hang up, I realized that maybe my father is calling me because he is lonely and wants my company too.

44

THE PSYCHIATRIST

As a young boy, my mother repeatedly told me that she was going to die. Whenever she had a headache, she complained of having a brain tumor. Whenever my head hurt, I imagined the same. My pain always went away, and I didn't die. But the thought of death stayed with me. I feared that when my work was finished, I would die. After every accomplishment, I knew that I would not survive to see the next one. Before getting on a plane, I'd tell my friends the location of my will, how to distribute my savings. And who would take care of my dog? At thirty-four, when I realized that I had been conscripted by my mother's fears and was not going to die, my life came crashing down because now I had to figure out how to live.

The walk from my office at the university to my house in the Saint Anthony Park neighborhood of Saint Paul was three city blocks. But on this particular summer evening when I left the building, my legs were heavy. I looked up. A blazing red sun was setting, and its heat was slowing me down, disorienting me. I wiped the sweat from my forehead. When I reached the corner, I stepped out in the road to cross the street. An approaching car blasted its horn. The warning sound rose in pitch as the car whizzed past. It came so close that the wind it carried pulled at my shirt. Only after reaching the end of the block did the driver let go of his horn. I stepped back on the curb and gave myself time to think about what I had just done.

This time I raised my eyes. I saw no approaching cars and crossed. I walked past two houses, paused, and looked up my front porch at the door. Climbing the steps, I began to cry. Halfway up, my book bag released from my grip. I let it fall. My hand trembled as I put the key in the lock and opened the door. By the time the front door closed behind me, I was sobbing profusely. My body jerked. My breathing was shallow. Between sobs, I gasped for air. I could not stop crying. Then I realized that maybe I shouldn't. This is what I should have done long ago.

On the outside, I was outgoing. But on the inside, I was alone. It was difficult for me to get out of bed in the morning to go to work. But once I was at work, I was fine. Day after day, I was cheerful at work, but once I started climbing the stairs to my house I started crying. At times, I was so remorseful I didn't want to live. Then I thought—who am I protecting and who should have protected me?

I wanted to get better. I didn't want to give up. I thought about those who helped me and who saw the value in me that I couldn't find in myself. What they saw was the determination and hard work handed down to me from my father, and the empathy and humility passed on to me from my mother. Those who cared for me were counting on me to care for myself. I didn't want to disappoint them, not the way my mother and father had disappointed me.

I read a lot: *Healing Your Aloneness,* by Erika Chopich and Margaret Paul; *Healing the Shame That Binds You,* by John Bradshaw; and feeling the forgiveness in the words of Elia Wise, who wrote *For Children Who Were Broken.*

I sought help from psychiatrists and psychologists. They prescribed Zoloft. My thinking became fuzzy, time slowed, and after a month of a dry mouth and diarrhea, I couldn't take it any longer and stopped the antidepressants. The doctors switched to trazodone. They said that it would help me sleep. But in the morning I was tired, and I was fatigued for the rest of the day. So I stopped that too. From then on, I knew that I had to do this without medication.

Every week, for a half hour, I met with the psychologist. I told him about my mother, her suicide, and my need for my father's love and approval.

At the end of each session, I'd ask, "What should I do?"

He never gave me a straight answer, but asked, "What do you want to do? How do you want to feel?"

At the end of the sixth session, we made a breakthrough. "I'm trying to make it work," I told him.

"Make what work?" he asked.

"My life," I answered. I opened one of my books, turned it sideways, and on a blank page drew a long line across the middle. On one end of the line, I wrote the word *TRUST,* and on the other end, the word *LOVE*. I pointed to the middle and asked, "How do I get this to work?"

He asked, "Can I give you a hug?"

I stood up and nodded. He walked from behind his desk and put his arms around me. I started to cry. I reached up and returned his hug, closing the gap between us. I knew that I was not alone and that I needed to stop isolating my feelings. I needed to be who I am, instead of what I thought my father wanted me to be.

My therapist said I want to put you in group therapy. I want to put you with other gay men.

What I thought that I was hiding, he knew the entire time. In retrospect, probably everyone else knew too.

In the beginning, it was easy for me to deny my sexuality. Or even that I had sex at all, which I hardly ever did, unless I count the solo acts of masturbation that made my life less hectic. Besides, as much as I wanted to be sexual, I was afraid of being that close to anyone. I had not learned how to be affectionate. I was afraid of letting anyone see who I really am. And no matter how well known I had become as a veterinarian or how proficient as an educator and caregiver, or how prominent my research was, it did not buffer me from imagining how devastated and hurt I'd feel if rejected. But what I was afraid of most, was telling my father that I was gay. It would be another chance for him to withhold his love. So I never came out to my father. Unable to gain his approval for the achievements of which I was proud kept me from telling him that I was gay, for which I was ashamed. I wanted to be the son my father would be proud of, so I ignored my feelings.

I avoided intimacy. Like my father, I kept everything bottled up, deep inside.

When I began venturing out on my own, it was disastrous. I couldn't tell the difference between flirting, sex, relationships, love, dating, or manipulation. And because I didn't have gay friends to help me sort it out, I was left with hurt and ambivalence. Maybe I had made the wrong choice. I retreated to my work and decided that rushing things and making up for lost time was a mistake. In a way, waiting was good. I was a teenager in the 1970s and a young man in the 1980s. Feeling unworthy of affection, I probably would have let things happen to me that I shouldn't. And at a time when AIDS was killing young gay men, I could have been one of them. I was celibate and emotionally immature, but I was healthy and alive.

45

JOE

I met Joe at the gym. He looked like my father, white, with a full head of dark-brown hair and a mustache. He played classical piano with the sensitivity of my mother. He liked movies and had a government job taking care of Minnesota's mainframe computers. He had started as a math major at the University of Minnesota in the 1970s but ended up in the theater. He was intelligent and politically opinionated but in a good way.

If you heard him tell the story of how we met, he would tell you that I was a stuck-up cat-piss doctor. He reminded me that whenever he tried to say hello, and he tried for months, I would look down at the floor and walk away. He sent Bill, one of his friends, over as a test to determine if I was friendly or not. Bill should have been in sales. He always smiled. He was a few inches shorter and a few years younger, but when he approached, his eyes widened and invited you in. When I stood up from taking a drink at the water fountain, Bill said hello. I can't remember what we talked about, the weather, our jobs, but it was friendly. It was like meeting someone pleasant in the checkout line at the grocery store. It was easy. I later heard that Bill reported back that I was not stuck-up. Of course, I was, and still am, a cat- and dog-piss doctor.

If you heard me tell the story, I would tell you that Joe was a stalker. During step aerobics class, if I looked past the glass wall, I would catch Joe staring at me. He had a work colleague trace my license plate number off my red pickup truck. Before I met Joe, he knew my name and where I lived.

I was surprised that I didn't see him at my job. Joe's cat had skin cancer from a leukemia vaccination and was being treated at one of the clinics at the veterinary hospital. His cat primarily saw oncology specialists. We never crossed paths because I was in internal medicine.

The day we finally did meet, he waited for me to strap myself into an exercise machine to work my legs. Getting into those machines was like preparing for an amusement park thrill ride. I climbed up into the seat, secured the front of my legs behind the tension bar, reached on my left and pulled up the seat belt, and snapped the end into the buckle. After he saw me locking myself in, Joe appeared wearing a blue T-shirt with the University of Minnesota's Raptor Center imprinted on the front. After a quick hello, he asked if I was familiar with the Raptor Center. I said yes, and that I worked at the veterinary hospital across the street. We talked about his cat, Tikki, and how Joe felt guilty. He thought that he was doing the right thing, protecting his cat from the leukemia virus by vaccinating him. I told him that he had done the right thing with the information that we had at the time. If I had my life to live over again, I would have made better choices too.

Our conversation veered to his older sister. I am not sure how we got there, but our words were serious, our eyes wider, and our voices muted. Joe's sister was dying of cancer. Doctors had misdiagnosed her pain. Instead of listening to her, doctors called her a hypochondriac; her husband had just been diagnosed with multiple myeloma. Her doctors told her that she "needed to relax." The doctors ignored her concerns until a lump surfaced near her clavicle. Her undiagnosed lung cancer had spread to her bones. She was in so much pain and regret for not insisting that her doctors do additional diagnostics that she asked Joe for help. She wanted Joe to find her a copy of the book, *Final Exit,* a suicide manual for those with a terminal disease. Joe's sister was contemplating suicide.

Even though it had been twenty-five years since my mother ended her life, the topic was still raw for me. I was reluctant to delve too much into his sister's anguish, since I harbored so much pain and loss that I had not resolved.

I took the position that suicide was wrong, that all life had a purpose. Sometimes the purpose is not obvious to the person considering the act. Maybe they serve as a role model to others. Joe's sister had three adult children. I could not imagine how they would cope with her loss. But I was being selfish. Still experiencing the pain of my mother's loss, I could not focus on how her family felt about her or her children and husband enduring the pain and suffering for an illness that was not going away. The one thing for certain is that she would die. And she did. Within a month, the tumor eroded into the vessels in her neck. She bled to death while choking on her own blood.

Even though the topic was heavy, being with Joe was easy. We talked for almost an hour. My workout? Well, let's just say it did not happen. Before leaving, I gave him my email address. The following Friday we made plans for dinner. I met him at a Chinese restaurant near his house. I am embarrassed to say this, but our first date lasted three whole days.

I didn't hide Joe from my father, but I was also not forthright with him. Joe and I traveled to Chicago several times to visit him. My father never asked about my relationship with Joe, and I never brought it up.

My father would die without knowing that I was in love and was being loved in return. But that was not his fault. I never told my father that I was gay, although I am sure that he knew. After graduating first in my class in veterinary school, I had earned a PhD and achieved specialist certification in internal medicine, but my relationship with my father was no better. I should have told him who Joe was. I still desperately wanted my father's love, and I was afraid that his disapproval of my relationship would be another strike against me.

46

CALL HOME

After eating dinner, I hear the phone ring. I reach for the receiver, but stop when I recognize the caller ID. It is my father again. I let the machine answer the call, but stand near to listen.

"Jody?" My father says as if he knew that I am listening. Then he repeats himself, "Jody, answer the phone." My father's voice is more insistent the second time.

Still, I do not answer the phone. I am not sure that I have the strength to tell him no again. My father and Gary need to solve their own problems. I stand closer and continue listening.

"Hello, Jody." His voice becomes more relaxed. "Anyway, Jody, this is your father. Give me a call when you get home. Okay, Jody? Okay, bye-bye." My father says call home one more time before he hangs up.

Three days later, on April 4, 2011, I am at work when my pager vibrates. Flashing on the green screen I read, "Your father is in the ER 773-259-6702."

I call the number right away. A nurse answers in the emergency room at the University of Chicago Hospitals. I tell her that I am returning a call and give her my name. She asks if Joseph Lulich is my father.

"Yes, what is wrong with him?" I said. I am speaking louder because I am worried.

"Your brother asked us to call you. He does not want to make any decisions about your father. I will find the doctor," the nurse said.

The neurologist in the emergency room informs me that when my brother brought in my father, he was incoherent and fading in and out of consciousness. Then the doctor completed the information with the diagnosis. "Your father had a stroke," the neurologist tells me.

I ask if they know the cause.

"Based on your father's age and heart disease, in all likelihood, it is a clot," says the neurologist.

"How long has he been hospitalized?" I ask.

"At least four hours," he says. "I am calling to ask if you want me to give medicine to break up the clot."

I didn't know what to do. My father hated hospitals. "That's where doctors kill you," he reminded me often. My father had just turned eighty-one, and although I had not been home in five years, I knew that he was slowing down. Without a definitive diagnosis, I made the decision that my father was too frail and had much to lose. I told the doctor no unless he thought that treatment would be overwhelmingly successful.

My father's stroke could not have happened at a more inopportune time for me. I had a two-hour lecture in about thirty minutes. The next morning, I had a 9:15 a.m. United Airlines flight to Washington, D.C. I was scheduled to provide two days of continuing education to veterinarians. But he was my father.

I called my brother. He said that Dad was sitting on the couch, and when he got up, he was unsteady and fell to the floor. "I rushed him to the hospital," Gary said. "He's quiet and stable now."

"I changed my flights," I told Gary. "I'll be home Thursday night after finishing my lectures in D.C. Please call me later tonight. I want to know how Dad is doing."

47

SAYING GOODBYE

When I walked into his hospital room, my father was asleep, resting on his side. The rising sun beamed through the window above his bed. It cast shadows over the floor of the swaying trees outside. The floor smelled like it had been recently mopped with the fresh scent of Spring Febreze. A smooth light-blue blanket covered him from the soles of his feet to the Adam's apple of his neck. His gray hair was tossed wildly over his head, long strands in one direction and shorter ones in another. His face was unshaven.

This was the bohemian father I grew up with. His scruffy appearance and unconventional social habits sometimes embarrassed me in front of my friends. He was health-conscious to the point of absurdity with his oregano oil, excessive garlic, no processed sugar, and his deep mistrust of the medical profession. He often scolded me and even my friends for any deviation of the slightest from his paragon.

As he lay there, I reminisced how he gently carried me in and put me to bed those many nights after returning home from the drive-in movies. I remember the spring of 1968, the day after Martin Luther King Jr. was assassinated. The streets in our neighborhood were erupting. Stores were looted and burning just two blocks from our house. My father walked through our predominantly Black neighborhood, picked me up from school, and walked me home. Being white, he took a big risk walking to pick me up at school. He could have been attacked. But he was not, and we both made it home safely.

I smiled as I looked down at him resting on his side. His eyes were closed and his breathing was easy. As I looked closer, his cheeks were sunken in, telling me that he was thinner than what I remembered.

I didn't want to wake him, but I wanted him to know that I was there. I leaned over and lightly rocked his shoulder. Dad, I said. Without opening his eyes, he shrugged his shoulder as if to motion me to leave him alone. Maybe he thought that I was the hospital staff. Maybe it was time for his medications. Finally, he opened his eyes but still did not look up. When he did, he squinted. He studied me. And when he recognized that it was me, he began wildly slapping my arms with floppy hands and pulling at my shirt sleeves. He tried to speak. His chest heaved up and down. But only raspy sounds came out as he forced air through an uncooperative larynx. I could tell that he was frustrated. His body was not doing what he told it to do. But he didn't have to say it, I knew that he was happy to see me.

It is okay, Dad, I said. He tried to speak again but mouthed unrecognizable syllables into unrecognizable words. He shook his head and lowered it in resignation.

I kept talking. I told him that I came straight from Washington, D.C., where I was lecturing. I told him about my dog at home, that his house was fine and that Gary, his eldest son, would be here soon. I talked and talked so that he did not have to. I talked until he calmed down. Then he sat up in bed, leaned forward, and lowered his head into his outstretched arms for me to come and sit next to him.

We never talked about this before. About what happens when life takes an uncertain turn. Having been ambushed by my mother's death, I wasn't sure that I knew how to begin this conversation either, so I skirted around it. I didn't want to talk about the possibility of my father dying even though I needed to know what he wanted me to do or not do now that he was in the hospital, now that he was old and frail, now that he was struggling to recover from a stroke.

In the past, when my father was sad or worried, he worked his way through it. Sometimes he wanted me near, and we worked our way through it together. We would go to the hardware store and buy nails or dry cement. We rebuilt the back stairs, or painted the kitchen blue, or laid a foundation for a backyard patio.

This was our awkward line of communication that we developed after my mother died. We avoided what mattered, but accomplished what the house needed, or the car needed, or what the tenants needed. He hoped and I hoped that time and working together would resolve what we both needed. For me it never did. My needs were not physical. I needed his love and his approval, not tasks. I needed his touch, and his smile and his shoulder, and his lap. I needed to know that he was happy and happy with me. I needed to know that he not only cared for me but cared about me. But he perceived it differently. After working on the house, or the car, or with the tenants, he had nothing left for me. Sometimes when he looked at me, I thought that he saw my mother and all the things that went wrong between them.

Now at eighty-one, he needed my help. And to make matters more difficult, the stroke took away his voice and maybe his reasoning. And like my father then, I lacked the emotional development and strength to comfort him now. I could ask about his illness and his prognosis. I could pull the blanket up over him if he was cold. I could be there for him, but I didn't know how to be there with him. It was difficult for me to be close to my father. There was so much pain between us that I didn't know how to love him without the past getting in the way.

I came to the hospital each morning and left in the evening, and the next evening and the one after that, being present, but not being there, not dealing with the possibility that my father may never come home.

When I visited Sunday morning, the day I was scheduled to fly home, my father's wrists were strapped to the railings on either side of his bed. The nurse told me that after I left the night before, he became agitated and pulled out his IV lines. He ran for the door, ran out of the room and down the hallway. When held back, he wailed and screamed and sat in the middle of the floor. To keep him from hurting himself, they had to restrain him, the nurse said.

Seeing him strapped to his bed was not the image I wanted to take with me before getting on the airplane. I asked them to undo the straps.

"I'll watch him," I told the doctor and the nurse.

It didn't take long for my father to realize that he had choices again, and he would use them. He quietly got out of bed. And before I realized what he was crafting, he swiftly grabbed the water bottle in the chair next to his bed and charged for the door. His hospital gown flapping in the wind revealed that he wore nothing underneath except a diaper. I stood up to stop him. He tried to run past me but instead ran into me.

Holding him back was not the solution. I opened my arms and hugged him. I held him while his feet still moved up and down, even though he went nowhere.

I pulled him in close. He smelled clean like sandalwood soap. I leaned my cheek into his. His short beard felt rough and prickly, but his skin was warm. I turned my face in his direction and whispered into his ear, "Dad, I love you." And with those words, time stopped. It was as if our relationship had a new reference point. The tension in his body vanished. He became quiet. He got it. He understood that I was there to support him. The water bottle he was holding fell from his hand and hit the floor, making a loud thud and sloshing sound as it rolled underneath the bed. He stopped running. But in one final attempt, he stood on the tips of his toes and fell into me. His left hand grabbed the back of my shirt and he held me tightly. He was unsteady but pulled himself closer. With his other hand balled into a tight fist, he gently rubbed the middle of my back.

At no other time did I feel more his son than I did then. At no other time did I regret not telling him sooner and more often that I loved him. My love was just love, free of the fear of rejection and uncomplicated by our history.

I wished I had extra sets of arms like Shiva the Hindu god of change, because everything had changed, and I held him tighter. I wanted my brother and the nurse and the doctor and anyone within arm's reach to be a part of this moment, this huddle of unconditional love and forgiveness. I pressed his head against my head, and his chest against my chest, and felt his heart beating against my beating heart. I wanted to take him home with me, but my father was too sick.

He couldn't feed himself. If my brother and I tried to feed him, we would risk food entering his lungs or suffocation.

The young nurse with a short Afro who watched the whole encounter seized the opportunity to clean up my father. She ripped apart the Velcro straps, dropping his soiled diaper to the floor. She flipped open the lid of the sanitary wipes, pulled up two, and wiped his butt and groin. She rushed to a side cabinet, grabbed a fresh diaper, and fastened it around his waist. With the skill of a basketball player, she flung the soiled diaper in one continuous arc from the floor, tossing it perfectly into the garbage can. It all happened so fast my father didn't budge. She looked up at me and nodded, and I winked, recognizing her orchestrated flair and alacrity.

With my arms still wrapped around my father, I moved him toward his bed, and he obliged. I lowered him in, pulled his gown down over his legs, and the blue blanket up to his shoulders. I leaned over and ran my fingers through his hair. In a soft voice, I reminded him that I had to leave soon, and in the same sentence told him that I would be back in a week. Summer was almost here, and I wouldn't have to teach until the fall. He smiled. I thanked him for being a good father, that I knew raising two young boys without a mother was difficult. I thanked him for not placing us in foster care. For giving me books and piano lessons. For teaching me how to work with my hands. I apologized for wanting more of him at times when he was busy or needed time for himself. And then I told him to not die on me.

48

REGRET

I flew back to Minnesota and was at work on Monday. I waited to hear how my father was doing, but no one called. Finally, that evening, I was able to get in touch with my brother, Gary.

"Dad is about the same," he said. They will anesthetize him to place a feeding tube tomorrow.

Tuesday morning as I drove to work, my cell phone rang.

"Is this Gary Lulich?" a hurried voice blurted.

"No, I'm his brother."

"This is the University of Chicago Hospitals. We anesthetized your father and placed the feeding tube. Immediately following the procedure his heart stopped. We're performing cardiac resuscitation, but I am afraid that there is little more that we can do. He is eighty-one years old. It's been over fifteen minutes. He's not responding. We are requesting permission to stop."

My eyes welled up. The traffic light turned green. The cars behind edged closer and then starting honking, ordering me to go forward. All I wanted was to go backward because I should have been there with him. I got back on the phone.

"No, I don't want him to die alone. Please don't stop! Call my brother."

"We tried calling your brother at the other number. No one answered."

Talking to myself, I wanted to scream. *Gary, don't let him die alone. You've got to get to the hospital. Dad is dying. Even if he's unconscious, he can still hear you. Tell him that we love him.*

But it was too late. Even if they contacted Gary, my brother lived fifteen minutes away. He would not reach him in time.

I pulled over to the side of the road with my phone still open and the nurse asking me what I wanted. As I shifted the gear in park, the first tear fell, and the second and the third and the twentieth and the hundredth. My vision blurred, and my eyes burned. I clutched the steering wheel as my head slowly lowered. My two dogs next to me in the passenger seat knew that I was losing it. The Chihuahua squeezed into my lap and rested between me and the steering wheel.

I didn't want my father to die alone. Not with someone pounding on his chest or breaking his ribs. Not with them shooting volts of electricity through his body trying to restart his heart, each volt contracting his muscles, jolting him up from his bed into the air. His face writhing in pain. His expression confused.

"Don't shock him," I pleaded.

Still unsure of my decision, I sat perfectly still. I hesitated. Then I said what I had hoped never to say. I said it so softly that I was not sure the nurse heard me. I said it softly because I couldn't bear hearing myself saying it, but I had to.

"Let him go. Stop. Just stop."

My father would die alone.

When I thought that I had nothing left in me, out poured the whimpering of loss and the wailing of regret. *Why wasn't I there? Why didn't I say no to the feeding tube? It was too late now.*

I hugged my dog as I imagined what the doctors were doing. I imagined them slowly stepping away from his hospital bed. They'd remove the oxygen mask, the ECG leads, and the pulse oximeter. They would turn off the monitors, and the room would become absolutely quiet because the absence of sound is what death must be like. Unfolding a clean white sheet, they would cover his feet and his legs, and then his waist and his chest, and his shoulders and his neck, and his chin, and his nose, and his eyes, and his tousled gray hair. They would turn the lights out, leave the room, and close the door.

49

———

LOST

I prayed that my father in his journey would not be alone. That he would find my mother.

Several years ago, my aunt Kathy, my mother's sister, came to visit after a long separation. There was so much I wanted to know about my mother.

"Am I like her?" I asked.

"Did she love us, my brother and me?"

"Did she ever say what she hoped of us when we grew up?" Like turning pages in a family photo album, we unfolded so many memories. Mine had many holes and places where pictures were missing. I had so many questions.

Then I asked my aunt Kathy if she would take me to my mother's grave, a place I had not visited since her death, not since I was nine years old. My father swore never to go back. We never went back to visit her grave, but I had too many questions to stay away. I needed to see where she was buried.

At first, my aunt agreed but later changed her mind. Burr Oak Cemetery, where my mother was buried, had been in the news. Burial plots were illegally resold. Caskets were buried one on top of the other. Lids of caskets were level with the earth. Some caskets were smashed and bodies wrongfully exhumed. Some remains were burned, and others buried just beneath the surface or dumped in a mound in a corner of the property. I wouldn't be able to find her, she said.

My mother was lost.

Dad, you need to find her. You need to find her because she may not recognize you. You've grown older and thinner. Your hair is gray, and you grew an untidy beard.

To find her, you'll have to recognize her gentle laughter, her warm touch, and her kind smile. To find her, you'll have to forgive her for her mistakes and understand that her alcoholism and her addiction to it were her disease, her call for help, her plea for love, her request to be held close.

After forty four years, I would have hoped that the animosity between them had shrunk into the tiniest of moments, small enough to fit on the head of a stick pin, and my father wearing his tan cashmere sports coat still too wide for his shoulders, white shirt, bronze tie, and gray slacks will take that stick pin and fasten a white cymbidium orchid to the lapel of my mother's muted pink dress that curved in slightly at her waist and curved out slightly at her hips before stopping just below her calves. He would gently reach forward and cup his hands around the back of her supple forearms, draw her in close, look deep into her eyes and smile, then slowly slide his hands down to meet her hands, clasp his hands around hers, use his thumbs to softly stroke the flesh between her thumb and first finger, then gently guide her hands behind his back to encircle his waist, drawing her in even closer. He would lightly kiss her lips, release the kiss, look deep into her eyes again, slightly cock his head to the right, and softly say, "I've missed you."

Will he find her?

He has to find her.

Because I couldn't.

50

GARY

One month after my father's death, a large white envelope arrived in the mail. I had been expecting it. I knew what was inside. I laid the envelope on the dining room table, pulled out a chair, and sat down. I hesitated. Then I broke the seal and removed a small stack of light-green, watermarked papers with the official state emblem in the lower left corner.

This was a first for me. I had never seen a death certificate. I gently ran my fingers over its surface. I anticipated that the papers would feel heavy and textured, but they were smooth and surprisingly ordinary. And yet, not being at the hospital when he died, this was my only tangible proof.

I started at the top and read every word.

Decedent's Legal Name, Joseph Lulich.

Date of Death, April 12, 2011.

Birthplace, Chicago, Illinois.

Marital Status, Widowed.

Father's Name, Samuel.

Mother's Name, Olga.

Method of Disposition, Cremation.

Cause of Death, Amyloid Cardiomyopathy.

Other Significant Conditions Contributing to Death. I paused. The entry was blank, but it should not have been. After his stroke, swallowing was difficult for my father. I worried that he might aspirate food into his lungs. Not being able to safely drink or eat was the one obstacle keeping him in the hospital, and he desperately wanted to go home. I approved the placement of a feeding tube. The three attending doctors, an Asian woman with short dark hair, a white man with light-brown hair, and a female East Indian medical student with thick black hair, tried to pass the tube down his nose. My father wailed in pain and pushed them aside. I asked them to stop and then agreed to a percutaneous feeding tube. It would go directly into his stomach and come out beneath the skin on the side of his abdomen. But it required anesthesia to place. Immediately after the tube was inserted, my father's heart stopped. If I had the chance to do it again, my decision would be different.

I lowered my head and closed my eyes. I could not read another word. I instantly became sad. I did not cry. I had done that weeks ago. But every indication of tears had not completely disappeared from my face.

But what I mostly felt was complete exhaustion. These papers carried the emotional weight of the relationship that I had with my father. And now, I needed these documents to close his accounts.

I called my brother to tell him that I had the certificates and that I was flying to Chicago next week. As usual, he didn't pick up the phone. I left the details on the answering machine and said that we should do this together.

When I arrived, Gary was standing in the front yard waiting for me. He was dressed like my father in gray cotton slacks and a dingy white work shirt. His clothes loosely draped his frame, exposing only his hands and face. As I moved in closer, no one could question that we were brothers. We had the same caramel-colored skin and dark-brown eyes. The same slim body and long oval face. The same stoic facial expression, a look of tentative fearfulness that I considered a lasting mark of an unpredictable childhood. When either of us smiled, there was an unmistakable trace of anxiety.

There were differences too. He was three inches taller and three years older. And if you looked closely, one of his fingers on his left hand had an oddly shaped nail, the result of a bicycling accident when he was a child. The tip of his finger was crushed when he curiously traced the inside edge of the bike chain as it meshed with the cogs of the sprocket wheel.

Seeing him, I tilted my head in the direction we needed to go. Together, we walked west into the afternoon sun and toward the neighborhood bank where my father kept his money. We never had much to say to each other before his death, and did not have much to say now. After closing the account, we walked to another bank. My father did not trust banks, or the government, or doctors. So he kept his money in more than one place and hid his heart from any medical professional and from us.

I asked Gary if Dad had a safe deposit box. He shook his head.

After closing all the accounts, I gave Gary half of the money and put the other half in a separate account to pay for the taxes and utilities on the house. We walked home in the same manner as we started, in silence and as if we did not know each other. But we were undoubtedly attached. Attached by a common bloodline and growing up in a dysfunctional family huddled together by suicide, abuse, and spotty parental oversight, not to mention the persistent animosity between the two of us.

Thankfully, I had arranged for a friend to pick me up and drive me back to the airport. I walked up the driveway, sat on the steps at the side entrance of the house, and waited. I thought Gary was going back inside. He didn't. He stood over me, blocking my view of the street. I looked his way several times, assuming that he had something to tell me. After what became an uncomfortable extension of silence, I looked at him and said, "Remember the time Dad brought home a monkey?"

"Yes, it was sad that the monkey did not live long," said Gary.

I felt the same.

"Remember the time Dad brought home Dorothy?" After saying her name, my mouth twisted to one side, indicating my disapproval.

"Yes, that was a mistake. I tried to forget her too," said Gary.

I agreed. She was a piece of work. One night she locked me in the basement until Dad came home. "I am going to miss him," I said.

"Who?" said Gary.

"Dad," I said. "He didn't always show it, but he loved us. Then again, there were times he put us through some unbelievable crap. Remember the time he toppled the kitchen table and smashed all of the dishes."

Gary looked away and said nothing.

"You mean you don't remember?" I said, questioning his body language.

Dad waited until two o'clock in the morning before pulling us out of bed on a school night. He made us stand at attention and told us not to lean on anything. When I rested my hand against the refrigerator, he snapped and told me to stand up straight. That was when Dad got up from the table and said, "When I ask you two to clean up your own mess, I mean it." And with one hand, he flipped the kitchen table in the air, tossing it on its side. The dishes on top fell to the floor and smashed into pieces. Then he took the clean dishes from the cabinets and one by one hurled them against the wall and the floor. I can still hear the sound of breaking glass and Dad screaming, "If you're not going to clean the dishes, then you don't need any." I half-smiled, thinking how ridiculous our father acted at times.

Gary furrowed his eyebrows. Then his gaze went over my head and up into the sky as if I were making all this up. Or as if he did not approve of me speaking authentically about our father.

"You mean you don't remember Dad smashing all the dishes in the middle of the night?" I said.

Gary answered so softly that I could hardly hear him.

I looked bewildered and cupped my left hand behind my left ear to catch his words

Seeing me do this, he straightened his back and clearly said, "No, I don't remember."

"What do you mean?" I said. I stood up and took my other hand out of my pocket. I looked up at Gary and said, "How about the time Dad slapped Mom and dragged her out the front door by her hair?"

He shook his head and said, "Dad would never hurt anyone unless he was provoked."

"Provoked," my voice loudly shrieked. "Dad was the abuser."

I could not believe what I was hearing. "Dad exploded that night because you refused to wash your dishes. You left them in the sink for days. I was tired of cleaning up your messes. I was done apologizing for things that I did not do." It was exhausting keeping the peace in our house.

With my eyes fixed firmly on Gary's eyes, I paused and then loudly gritted out, "If Dad was so perfect, who taught you to hit our mother? And to hit me?" The birds overhead in the tree flew up into the sky. A little boy skipping down the sidewalk stopped and looked up the driveway. I stared back at him, and he quickly continued on his way. I leaned forward and waited for Gary to answer. The silence between us was long and thick and full of resentment. But I did not back down. I wanted an answer.

A single bead of sweat starting at the hairline slid down the side of my brother's face. The heat affected me too. I could feel myself boiling over. That was when a black SUV pulled up close to the curb. The passenger window lowered. "Jody, are you ready to go?" said Kenny Galvin in a welcoming voice. I was ready to go all right. I reached down and whisked up my backpack. Without saying a word, I shook my head as I walked past Gary. *Just let it go,* I told myself. I got in the car, closed the door, and as we drove away, I did not look back.

51

THE AWARD

After my father's death, work had little purpose. When he was alive, I had the momentum to always do my best. I worked hard because of him. He saw value and honor in my ability to help animals, even though he didn't always approve of my methods. I had been trained in traditional Western medicine. After he became a vegetarian, and a proponent of herbalism and colloidal metal therapy, he disagreed with my approaches. But he was my father, and no matter how old I was, I still wanted his approval. I loved him, and I needed him to love me back. Now that he was no longer alive, my interest in work deteriorated.

At a time when I was feeling more lost than ever, my cell phone rang. That was when Dan called. When he told me that I had been awarded the prestigious Mark Morris Lifetime Achievement Award. Dan explained that the award would be presented in one month at the North American Veterinary Conference and emphasized that it would be a great honor to see me accept the award, especially since he would be the one presenting it to me. That was when Dan worried that I would not show up. What he didn't know was why.

When I graduated from high school, I pleaded with my father to attend the ceremony. My father never finished high school. I was graduating with honors. I assumed that he'd be proud of me. I was excited about the opportunity for him to meet my teachers and hear what they had to say about me. When he didn't show up, I felt worthless. I questioned why life was so difficult and why I worked so hard. If not for the Galvins hooting as I walked across the stage to receive my diploma, I am not sure that I would have made it home that night.

My father was not all bad. When I needed help building science projects, he'd lend a hand and an opinion. Seeing me struggling through math and chemistry problems at the kitchen table, he'd deliver a pat of encouragement on my shoulder. I learned that he appreciated the journey more than the reward at the end. Maybe that explained why he missed all my graduations and every award ceremony. Needless to say, I began to feel the same. I paid less attention to graduations and skipped award ceremonies. However, I promised Dan that I would be at this one. Now that the date was close, I wished that I had not made the commitment.

Two days before the ceremony, I boarded the plane in Minneapolis on my way to Orlando, Florida. I didn't want to do this alone. Joe boarded the plane with me. I reached between our seats, grabbed the end of the seat belt, and inserted it into the buckle. It fastened with a loud click. I bit down on my lower lip and let out a low, nervous sigh, forcing the air out through my nose.

Joe looked over at me and said, "Are you okay?"

I nodded.

"What are you going to do?" he said.

"What do you mean?"

"You know what I mean. Your acceptance speech. Are you going to tell them your story?"

"I don't know. Do you think that anyone really cares?"

"Whatever you decide, it will be great," he said. "You'll do fine."

But I wasn't fine. I promised Dan that I would be there. And now I wished I hadn't.

I stuffed my backpack under the passenger's seat in front of me, but I couldn't take my eyes off it. Although I had mulled over my acceptance speech in my mind, I had written only a few key words and short phrases. There was still a lot of work to do.

Passengers continued to board the plane. I reached down, unzipped the top compartment of my backpack, pulled out a legal-size pad of yellow paper, and began to write.

I want to thank those who nominated me. No, that's not what I want to say. I was thankful for those who nominated me, I guess, but I didn't want to start this way. I tore off the sheet and started again.

Greetings from Minnesota, where our winters are cold, but our hearts are warm. Yuck. Sounds like I'm writing a travelogue. I drew a line through that one.

Serving the profession had been a joy and a privilege. Sounds good, but I didn't completely believe that. Why did I write it in the past tense? I will leave it and edit it later.

Receiving this award is an honor. Mmm. First humbled and now grateful, I liked these two sentences together.

Then I wrote, *Let me tell you why.* Am I really going to do this? Tell them why?

When I was nine years old, my mother . . . I stopped writing. I couldn't finish it. It didn't matter: the speech had been in my head all month, and my story had been buried in me for forty-six years.

The lights on the plane flickered off and on. Gusts of cold air spewed from the vent over my head. I drew myself inward to keep warm. I squeezed my knees together and began to tremble.

The engines roared and the plane jerked as it accelerated down the runway. That initial thrust forward slid me backward. My head pressed against the back of the seat. The plane shook and rumbled as we sped faster and faster down the runway. The nose of the plane pitched up. I held on to the armrests. The wheels lifted from the tarmac. I sank deep into my seat as gravity, the plane's upward trajectory, and my regret pulled my body down, struggling to free itself from the appearances that for such a long time kept me grounded. Now airborne, the plane arched on an eastward path. The left wing dipped. Through the window, I saw the snow-covered lakes and skyscrapers of Minneapolis behind us. Our next stop would be Orlando.

52

———

THE VENUE

When the plane landed in Orlando, it was already dark. We picked up a rental car and made the thirty-minute drive to the hotel.

The Gaylord Palms hotel is immense. Reminiscent of a grand Floridian mansion, its Spanish colonial revival architecture with low-pitched roofs and smooth beige terra-cotta plaster was like a ghost calling us back in time. We drove the car through the gate and followed the curved driveways past the large portico. We avoided driving up to the main entrance and instead parked the car off to the side and wheeled our luggage up the long driveway and walked in. Dark-brown leather chairs, wrought iron railings and balconies, and stone floor tiles created an old-world Spanish decor throughout the entrance. Farther inside, a large atrium filled with palm trees, stone grottoes, and an artificial waterfall and stream greeted us. Nine stories above a glass-and-steel dome connected all the buildings. The symmetry of the glass roof with its outward branching beams and crisscrossing steel lace was spectacular but resembled a spider's web. I began to feel uncomfortable. Tomorrow's ceremony would take place at the opposite end of the complex in a large auditorium.

We checked in. Our room was on the third floor. We walked in, and I turned on my computer. I was sure that I would have a message from Dan. And indeed, I did.

"Jody, let's meet in the afternoon, around 1:30. I can show you the auditorium, and we can talk about plans for the evening. There are others getting awards and you will be near the end."

In the space below, I typed "see you at 1:30 pm," and sent the message on its way.

When I arrived the next day, Dan was running around with a wireless microphone clipped on behind his head and over his ear. A flesh-colored extension with a tiny microphone on the end came from behind his left ear and extended out in front of his mouth. "Testing one two three, testing one two three," he repeated as he walked from one side of the stage to the other. His voice was clear, in command, and echoed in the empty auditorium. When he looked up, he saw me standing at the back entrance. He shouted, "Come up here, I want to show you what the stage feels like."

The stage was on three-foot risers and thrust out into the audience's seating. There were seats for over a thousand. They were arranged in multiple sections around the stage.

I walked up the middle aisle. When I reached the stage, Dan motioned me to the left and pointed to the stairs. "Come up on this side," he said. You will be seated in the audience near these stairs. "I want you to know where to enter because it may be dark. But when you come up, we will make sure to shine a spotlight on you."

Hearing that made me nervous. I walked up the stairs and hesitantly placed my left foot on the stage.

"Don't worry," he said. "It will be simple. I will introduce you. You will come up. The mic will be upfront. I will hand you the award. You will have about fifteen seconds to say thank you to the audience. Then you can take your seat. After the awards, we have a comic and a band for entertainment."

I was still stuck on the fifteen seconds. Which speech do I say? Maybe I should just say thank you. Short and simple. I looked at Dan, and my eyes opened wide.

"What?" Dan said. "Are you okay?"

I nodded twice. "I think so."

The last thing Dan said was, "We have a camera crew. They are not up yet, but large TV screens will be strategically placed around the stage like a rock concert. Images of your face and members of the audience will be projected around the room, on the sides, and over the top of the stage. We want the audience to be a part of the event. We want them to see and feel the excitement of everyone attending."

I half-smiled and said, "Brilliant." But less enthusiastically than what he expected. The more Dan revealed, the more I felt exposed. I turned around and made my way to the back of the stage. I walked down the stairs and toward the door that I came through. On the way out and from the back of the hall, I waved and shouted, "See you in a few hours."

He shouted back, "Come in the far-right door and we will let you in early before the crowd."

The door closed behind me.

Phew! My lips formed a tight circle as I exhaled. I loosened two more buttons on my shirt to cool down. I knew that it was going to be difficult. But I also knew that I still had a choice.

I walked across the courtyard to my section of the hotel complex. The elevator came right away. I pushed the button for the third floor and went back to my room. I unlocked the door and threw myself across the bed. I wanted to rest and so did my body, but my mind raced. It tumbled back and forth between the two versions of my speech. *Who cares why I became a veterinarian?* Besides, most of the audience will attend for the entertainment.

53

HOURS TO GO

That morning, Joe left for Disney World, promising not to miss the event. I handed him the ticket to get in and said see you tonight.

Hours before the ceremony, I stood in the middle of my hotel room, alone, wearing a white T-shirt, boxer briefs, and black socks pulled up to the calves. I took a deep breath through my nose and emptied it into my mouth. My cheeks filled like balloons. Then the air gushed out, flapping my lips, sounding like a whinnying horse. I quickly covered my mouth with my hands and, in doing so, tasted the salt from the sweat on my palm. Did I want the audience to know that my mother was an alcoholic and committed suicide? That I became a veterinarian not out of compassion but out of heartbreak and obligation?

I'm keeping my promise. I'm here, even though telling the truth is what I feared the most.

I opened my luggage and took out my dark-blue suit. I laid it across the bottom of the bed. With my hands, I slowly smoothed out the wrinkles from being folded and packed. That suit and how I cared for it reminded me of how my education and career afforded me the opportunity to lecture around the world: Japan, New Zealand, Africa, Australia, and many countries throughout Europe.

I sat on the edge of the bed, stretched my arms over my head, and lay back. I couldn't relax. I got up. I unzipped the front pocket of my backpack and pulled out my speech. I read it and then plopped down into a dark-brown leather chair next to the bed. I sunk in deep. The leather was cool and stuck to my bare thighs. I leaned forward, set the speech on the desk, pulled the chair up close, and read the speech again. Then I turned it over. I grabbed a pencil and began writing a new speech, one less revealing.

On behalf of the teachers and mentors who guided me, and the clients and patients who trusted and appreciated my care, I accept this prestigious award in their honor. It has been my goal to teach my students as I wished to be taught and to care for my patients as I would want to be cared for. I thank the committee for selecting me. It's an honor to be acknowledged by your peers.

The writing came easy. An alternate speech was something I had considered from the start. But this one needed a better opening.

I became a veterinarian because the doctor who cared for my sick dog was gentle and kind. At a young age, I knew I wanted to be just like him. That's it, I thought. *That's all they need to know. It wasn't the truth. But it was what I had been telling all these years.*

I got up from the desk, entered the bathroom, and shaved. I stepped over the rim of the tub into a pounding hot shower. I turned around and leaned my back into the spray. My muscles relaxed. My breathing slowed. The bathroom filled with steam, and I was becoming invisible.

I stepped out of the tub and toweled dry. I slipped my arms into the sleeves of my white shirt and fastened the buttons. I stepped into my trousers, pulled them up, closed the clip at the waist, and lifted the suspenders up onto my shoulders. After twenty years, the pants still fit. I flipped my shirt collar up and placed my necktie underneath it. I fashioned a half-Windsor knot. The silk slid effortlessly over my fingers. I pushed the knot up to my neck, closed the top button on my shirt and the smaller ones fastening the points of my collar over the tie. I donned my jacket and secured the middle button. I looked in the mirror. I lifted my chin. I smiled. I admired how confident a change in clothes made me feel. I was ready to give either speech but had to decide which one. I turned the lights off in the room, closed the door behind me, and took the elevator down to the main floor.

When I arrived, the auditorium was locked. A small crowd huddled around the entrance. They joked with one another while waiting for the doors to open. Their laughter put me at ease.

One of the organizers poked her head out of a side door. She recognized me and waved me over. She put her hand on my shoulder, stepped to the side, and led me in.

Workers in blue vests and headsets darted back and forth checking the setup of the room. One carried a thick cable to a large video camera on a tripod in the center. Another video camera was on a riser in the back, and a third one was onstage. A voice in the back shouted out, "Camera one." A large screen at the back of the stage lit up and projected a view from the audience. "Camera two." An image cutting across the stage from left to right filled the screen. "Camera three." Five additional screens circling the back and sides of the auditorium lit up. Camera three was the one on the riser in the back. It focused on the stage and then zoomed in and out, enlarging and shrinking the picture. Then all the screens went dark, and the hall was quiet. My footsteps echoed against the concrete floor as I made my way up front and to my seat. I glanced at the sheet of paper dangling from my hand. On one side—the invisible speech. On the other side—the truth. I turned the paper over and over. I needed to decide.

With sudden synchronicity, the four entrances to the auditorium opened simultaneously. The heavy metal doors made loud thuds as they hit the stops bolted on the floor that latched them open. The lights came up over the audience. Attendees made their way up the aisles in waves. They stopped to acknowledge old friends and introduce new ones. They greeted one another with handshakes and hugs. The chatter that was once outside was now bubbling inside. Lights at the back of the stage went from soft amber to bright beams of red, green, and blue. Tall speakers on either side filled the room with rhythmic upbeat music.

I looked around. Many faces I knew. Many I did not. The incoming audience made me nervous. Time moved quickly. I was excited but worried. I see Joe, front row and center. He had his high-definition video camera poised and ready to film every word. If Grace were alive, she would sit next to him, place her hand over his, and squeeze it lightly in recognition of what was about to happen. I looked up at the ceiling and smiled in case she was watching. With the auditorium almost full, I turned back around and sat down in my seat.

My thoughts returned to my mother's death. *If I knew then what I know now, I would have stopped her. I did not know that antifreeze would kill her. I did not know that her kidneys would shut down and that she would suffer. I did not know that the hospital would refuse her dialysis because the technology was scarce, and an attempted suicide excluded her from treatment. I did not know that there was a window of opportunity, in which the antidote if administered within hours would prevent serious harm. I did not know that losing her would be so painful. How could I have known? I was only nine. But if I knew, I would have knocked the glass out of her hand. I would have called for an ambulance. I would have run out that evening and found my father.*

The lights go down over the audience and up on the stage.

54

THE SPEECH

The lights onstage intensify. The music swells. The announcer strolls up from the back of the stage. Applause fills the auditorium. He grabs the microphone and brings it close to his mouth.

Suddenly, my thoughts turn inward. *What would the audience think if I tell them that both my parents were alcoholics? That my mother committed suicide? That my father was physically abusive and beat her? Good or bad, these are the events that shaped who I am. I hadn't made up my mind yet. But I need to decide soon. Which speech do I tell?*

The music dies down. The bright lights dim. A spotlight focuses on the emcee. I hear laughter and then more applause, but my attention now zeroes in on the sheet of paper in my hand. I fold it. I open it up. I turn it over. I read it again, and this time close my fist around it.

I won't need this sheet of paper if all I am going to do is accept the award and say thank you. But just saying thank you is not who I am, and not who I want to be. *My career and this award were carved out of the hardships and dysfunctions of my family. Or was it? If it wasn't, then how did I get here? If it wasn't, then why am I being honored?* Immediately after that thought, the emcee brings up the next award.

A large screen over the stage ignites in blue with a black silhouette of a man and his dog. I know that image. It's a silhouette of me. I'm sitting on a park bench. My eight-year-old Dalmatian, Max, is leaning against my knee.

Dan, the veterinarian who called me a month ago to make sure that I attended the ceremony, has the honor of introducing the award.

"The Mark L. Morris Lifetime Achievement award is presented to an individual who has made a lifelong commitment to improving the health and well-being of companion animals." Dan continues, "This year's recipient is a professor of internal medicine at the University of Minnesota. His work in nephrology and urology has earned him an international reputation as a clinical investigator and educator. He is codirector of the Minnesota Urolith Center. He created voiding urohydropropulsion, a nonsurgical technique to rapidly remove urinary stones. The winner of this year's prestigious award," Dan pauses, "is Dr. Jody Lulich."

I hear loud applause. A spotlight shines in my direction. It follows me as I stand up and make my way up the stairs from the side of the stage. When I reach center stage, Dan's smile beams and he hands me the award. It's a bronze statue of Dr. Mark Morris with his dog at his side. My name is embossed on the front of its base. I had not anticipated its weight. It dips slightly as he hands it to me. I lift it up to view and then show the audience.

Dan approaches the microphone, "In recognition of Dr. Lulich, Hills Pet Nutrition will donate twenty thousand dollars to the Morris Animal Foundation in his name."

I hand the award back to Dan and approach the microphone. I smile and face the crowd. I notice that my image and every word that I am about to say is being broadcast on multiple screens that circle the perimeter. I am conspicuously surrounded by myself. I hesitate and then lean into the microphone.

This is truly an honor, I tell them.

Let me tell you why. I entered this profession under not so usual circumstances. Yes, I care about animals. Yes, I get excited about science and discovery and medicine.

I pause and think about what I am going to say next. When I begin, my voice is shaky. My pace is deliberate. And my tone is somber.

Let me tell you why.

When I was nine years old, my mother perceived that her life was unbearable, and committed suicide.

The audience is silent. I don't tell them that my mother killed herself by drinking antifreeze. I don't mention that I was in the room watching her as she drank it. I don't tell them that although I did not know what antifreeze was, I knew that she was hurting herself. I do not tell them that I did not call for help.

I continue.

Two days later my mother died. My father, while driving my brother and me to her funeral, ran over a dog.

I hear someone in the audience gasp, but I know that if I stop, I might not be able to finish. I keep speaking

My father must have thought that my brother and I had suffered enough. He chooses not to stop the car and not to help the dog. We keep driving. What he does not realize is that I would carry the image of that injured dog with me for the rest of my life. Not only the pain that the dog endured but the pain of that dog's family when they discover that their dog, their beloved pet, has been mortally injured. I vowed to make it better. Despite such horrific beginnings, I am fortunate. I am fortunate because my journey has been filled with so many caring people guiding me . . .

I mention Grace Hooks, Carl Osborne, others, and continue:

and the many dogs and cats who needed my help.

My chest fills with air entering through my nose with an audible rush. I must have forgotten to breathe. I notice that my gaze has dipped from the audience to the floor of the stage. I straighten my back, lift my head, and look at the audience again. My voice tapers but I remember to be strong.

Let me tell you a story about one of those dogs. Kippy, a miniature schnauzer, was one of my first patients. He is a beautiful young dog. He developed acute kidney failure. His disease is so severe that his kidneys have shut down and he is not making urine. His prognosis is poor.

I still do not tell them that my mother died from acute kidney failure from drinking antifreeze.

Kippy is in ICU, hooked up to IV lines and other tubes.
His owners come to visit. They make a simple request. "Can we take Kippy for a car ride?" Initially, I hesitate. Kippy is very sick. But I agree to a short car ride. I watch them as they drive off. They leave in a white convertible. The top is down. As they pull out of the parking lot, I see Kippy lifting his head, catching the breeze. They are back in an hour. Kippy returns with more life in him than I have seen with all of my treatments. His owners are effusively grateful for the time with him.
Kippy returns to ICU. I hook him back up to his intravenous fluids. And within hours and for the first time in days, his kidneys begin to make urine. Not a little, but a lot. Within a few days, Kippy makes a complete recovery. What becomes very clear is that veterinary medicine is more than curing disease. It is about listening. Listening to what is important in life. It is about healing, healing the patient, and healing the hearts and minds of the patient's family.

My voice is somber again, but as I continue, it becomes stronger.

Unbeknownst to my clients, as I helped them, they were helping me heal. By accepting this award, I pledge to continue my journey of healing by making a compassionate difference in the lives of my patients, their families, my students, and my fellow colleagues.

I set it free. My struggle. My shame. Her death. My father's mistakes. My mistakes. And my efforts at keeping that part of my life a secret.

I lean back into the microphone, softly clear my throat, pause, and say, "Thank you."

My final words echo through the auditorium as if no one were out there. There is silence. I begin to shudder. I slowly turn around and start the lonely walk to the back of the stage. With each step, I question if I did the right thing. I can hardly lift my feet. My mind fills with regret. The bright lights shining from the back of the stage are blinding me, making it difficult for me to see where I'm going. I lower my head, but keep walking.

Then I hear clapping, muffled at first. It starts from the back of the auditorium. Then within seconds a few more and a few more. Suddenly, the clapping swells as it moves toward me like a wave filling the auditorium. One person stands. Then another, and another. I turn around and walk back to the microphone.

I am overwhelmed. I did not expect this to happen. I take in a deep breath and muster all of my strength to not cry. I look out in the audience. A wide smile replaces my ambivalence. They are giving me something that I have not had in a long time—a sense of acceptance.

In the back of the auditorium, I see a middle-aged man, dark hair, beige sports coat. He claps, not fervently like the rest of them, but with the steady beat of a slow march. I struggle to focus. The edges become sharper as my vision works its way inward. *Dad? Impossible. He has been dead for almost a year.*

I am haunted. Haunted by the need to be loved. To know that I belong to someone. To know that I belong here. So I lose myself in the alchemy of it. I wander through the muck of the now and of my past, of the living and the dead, of the answers and the unanswerable.

Is he really standing? He rarely showed his approval and even less his affection. Was withholding his love a way to draw me in close without losing control over me? Or was he afraid of allowing himself to love me, knowing how painful it would be if he lost me? Maybe that's why I felt alone when I was with him. Maybe that's why the more I tried to please him, to love him, and to get him to love me back, the more I lost him. I am losing him now. His face disappears into the audience.

I close my eyes and ask myself—*Was it all worth it? I could have given up. I almost did.*

My answer is clear. When I am feeling capable and distracted by the needs of others, so much so that I can let go of my own feelings and contribute to the success of those around me, I feel great. These are the times I live in my achievements and not my failures.

But when I am alone, or think about my childhood, or at Christmas, or when I struggle to fall asleep at night, or when I stay in bed too late in the morning, that's when it, the darkness, finds me. That's when I realize that in the past, my mother's earlier attempts at suicide were always thwarted because as a family we worked together. We pulled her through it no matter how forcefully she kicked at us, or spat on us, or tried to run away. As a family, we all understood not to let go of her. And when it was all over, she was loving and remorseful and thankful. And made the most delicious dinners, and laughed at our foolishness, and played piano and hummed while cleaning the house, and in the evenings read us stories that set our sleep into wistful imaginings of resolution and forgiveness.

But, this one time, we failed.

No, I cannot be faulted with giving her the momentum to rise up through her despair, walk in the kitchen, fill a glass with antifreeze, and drink it. Neither can I be faulted with the abrupt disappearance of my father, whose anger and disgust hurled him past his threshold of caring and, instead of being there, walked out the front door when he was needed most.

Then I realize my part. I was silent. However passive or thoughtful, I kept it a secret and told no one until it was too late to save her.

What I am left with—is remembering. Remembering, that when I was nine years old, my mother committed the ultimate act of selfishness by taking her own life. I will never know if it was a cry for help, an act of bravery, a strategic miscalculation, or mental illness. I knew that she was immensely sad. And I know that somewhere deep in the recesses of my consciousness still lives a heartbroken nine-year-old child who will forever regret his selfless act of silently letting her go while believing he was loving her.

The audience comes into view. My head slowly lifts as if perfectly hinged between my shoulders. Tears are welling up in my eyes. I blink furiously. Then I open my eyes and focus. Everyone is standing. Their loud clapping and appreciative rumbling crests—and jolts me back to the present. The ground beneath my feet is firm. I know where I am. I know why I am here. *And I am not alone.*

EPILOGUE

After that night and for years to come, I realized that telling the truth was the best decision. It freed me. Receiving the award and the audience's response told me that I belong here. When I teach my students about the dog with the green vomit who dies of acute kidney failure, I no longer keep it a secret and tell them why this lecture is so important for me. I tell them that my mother committed suicide by drinking antifreeze. I tell them that if I knew then what you now know, we could have saved her. The pain of hearing those words causes me to pause. When I continue, I look into their eyes and tell them, "By teaching you, her death has new meaning for me." Hearing this, the class is silent. They understand that the lesson is more than a lecture about kidney disease. They recognize that it is also a lesson about life and finding purpose.

*

In the spring of 2017 with my father's ashes in my backpack, I took a morning flight to Chicago and drove the rest of the way to Burr Oak Cemetery. Months earlier, I had found my mother's grave. Unlike so many plots in Burr Oak that were desecrated, dug up, or double-stacked, my mother's grave had not been disturbed. Her burial plot in section six, lot eleven, row thirty-eight was safe, but only a small metal plot number staked to the ground identified the spot. I didn't want to lose her again. I immediately ordered a pink granite grave marker.

When I arrived, I got out of the car and walked the gravel path as it meandered through an open field of thick grass and few trees. Flat grave markers dotted the landscape. Dark green moss anchored itself over the names of the deceased. I stayed on the path until the map indicated that I needed to walk over grass. I knew that I was close when I spotted a muted pink grave marker among the other weathered gray stones.

With less than twenty feet to go, my pace slowed. I was losing it. My eyes were wet with tears. When I reached her grave, I dropped to my knees. The ground was cold. The morning dew seeped through the knees of my pants and clung to my skin, connecting me to her. I kept still. I let the earth above her feel my weight. I wanted her to know that I had finally come to visit.

The journey had been long. It took me fifty years to arrive at the place that marked the separation between the nine-year-old boy remembering his mother's love before her death and the man I am today. I just kept thinking through all the possibilities. If I had acted differently, would she be alive?

I leaned over and touched the stone. It was cold. I took my finger and passed it over the grooves spelling out her name. BETTY JEAN LULICH. And read the words inscribed: COMPLICATED AND MIS-UNDERSTOOD, BUT ALWAYS LOVING.

I slipped off my backpack and set it on the ground. I opened it and removed a small garden shovel. At the foot of her tombstone, I began digging a hole. After it was almost a foot deep, I used my hands to excavate more soil. Reaching in, I pulled up rich black dirt. The

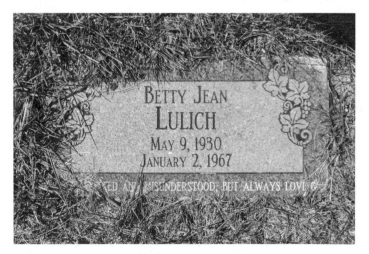

Mother's gravestone

moist earth collected underneath my fingernails and seeped into the cracks of newly broken skin. When done, I reached in my backpack again. This time I pulled out a brown cloth sack. Inside was a clear plastic bag with my father's ashes. I opened the bag and poured his ashes down the hole. A plume of his remains rose up in front of me. When it settled, I pushed the excavated dirt back into the hole and mounded the soil over the spot.

Perhaps my mother would not be happy with what I've just done. In many ways, she was running away from her marriage. In the end, they are together just as I always wanted them to be.

I opened a packet of marigold seeds and spread them over the bare earth in front of her grave. I emptied my water bottle and moistened the ground to give the seeds a growing chance. Marigolds are hearty, I told myself. They will flower and reseed themselves.

ACKNOWLEDGMENTS

I thank you, Loft Literary Center of Minneapolis. I did not have the confidence that I could complete a book until the center awarded me the Mentor Series. The teachers and other winners nourished me for a year and beyond. I was so excited after I completed my first draft but fully understood that a book comes alive in the process of revision. My work blossomed with the guidance and encouragement of Laura Shaine Cunningham, Mary Carroll Moore, Carolyn Holbrook, and my writing group.

JODY LULICH is a professor of veterinary medicine at the University of Minnesota. He is a renowned educator, clinician, and researcher and has written more than four hundred publications in scientific journals and books. He is a classical pianist, lectures around the world, and lives in the Twin Cities with his husband, Joe Linn.